Praise for *Next*

"I LOVE THIS BOOK! It will make you laugh, and perhaps make you cry a little. But whatever stage of the 'romance life cycle' you find yourself in, Barbara Summers' excellent advice, practical tips, and her insights into male and female behavior will encourage and inspire you to take the next steps toward a more joyful intimate life. I never thought I'd dip my toes back into the dating waters, until I laughed and cried my way through *Next!*

—Anne Doyle
Author of *POWERING UP! How America's Women Achievers Become Leaders*

"This fun, motivational book gives nuggets of practical advice that are soundly grounded in psychological principles. Every woman should read it."

—Richard Levak, PhD
Del Mar Clinic
Del Mar, California

"Most of us have experienced Mr. Wrong and looking for Mr. Right. *A Matchmaker's Guide to Finding Mr. Right, Ditching Mr. Wrong, and Everything In Between* is enlightening and brings us back to the basics of the real way to manifest Mr. Right and not settling for less than you want. It encourages you to have faith in yourself, to leave behind the desperation of meeting someone, and just letting fate happen. Barbara's book has the recipe for a successful relationship. Enjoy the read!"

—Jaki Baskow
President of Baskow and Associates, Las Vegas, Nevada
www.baskow.com
Proud Winner of DMC Partner for five years in a row
Recognized as Small Business of the Year by the Las Vegas Chamber of Commerce
Featured as "Queen of Las Vegas" in *Bel Air Magazine*

"There are many choices to take and directions to turn in life. This book helps you take the leap and make life happen. *Next!* will help you reflect on your relationships and ensure you're living abundantly in a vibrant and healthy relationship. It's a dynamic read for any stages of your relationship. An absolute must-read!!"

—Lane Ethridge
Founder Changing Lanes International

Next!

Next!

A Matchmaker's Guide to Finding Mr. Right, Ditching Mr. Wrong, and Everything In Between

BARBARA SUMMERS
with Carey Blakely

SelectBooks, Inc.
New York

This edition published by SelectBooks, Inc.
For information address SelectBooks, Inc., New York, New York.

First Edition

ISBN 978-1-59079-293-3

Library of Congress Cataloging-in-Publication Data

Summers, Barbara, [date]
  Next! : a matchmaker's guide to finding mr. right, ditching mr. wrong, and everything in between / Barbara Summers with Carey Blakely. -- First Edition.
      pages cm
  Summary: "Professional matchmaker and relationship coach, who is responsible for hundreds of women and men finding their marriage partners, gives advice on successful dating, finding love, keeping the spark in marriage, leaving failing relationships, and healing after divorce. She draws from experiences of her several marriages and tells stories of the singles she has matched"-- Provided by publisher.
  ISBN 978-1-59079-293-3 (pbk. : alk. paper) 1. Dating services. 2. Interpersonal relations. I. Blakely, Carey. II. Title.
  HQ801.S9268 2015
  302--dc23
                    2014032749

Book design by Janice Benight

Manufactured in the United States of America
10 9 8 7 6 5 4 3 2 1

*To my mother, whose strength has always inspired me
and who has stood by my side through the good and the bad.*

*And to my husband, Robert, who believed in my vision for this book
and helped make it a reality.*

Acknowledgments

I would like to thank Carey Blakely, my writer, for the joy she brought me during our collaboration. Her sense of humor and creativity made the journey a true pleasure.

I am also grateful to Rachel Thomas for her enthusiastic support and for taking the crucial step of introducing me to Eugene (Gene) Schwartz, which sent *Next!* on its way to publication. Likewise, I am indebted to Gene for rallying behind the concept and first draft and then introducing us to literary agent William (Bill) Gladstone of Waterside Productions. Bill's go-get-'em attitude and industry insight kept *Next!* in motion, and I thank him for his stellar work in securing a book deal. That brings me to the talented team at Select-Books, Inc., whose endeavors as a publishing company brought *Next!* into its final, fine-tuned form as an actual book. Thanks especially to Kenzi, Nancy, and Kenichi Sugihara for their hard work and publishing expertise! Finally, I express a heartfelt appreciation to my family for their love and support.

Contents

Next!

Introduction

Are you tired of being single? Are you ready to find someone new?

*Do you want to bring the excitement back into
a relationship that's lost its sparkle?*

Are you scared to leave a marriage that isn't working?

WHETHER YOU ARE A WOMAN LOOKING for a relationship, presently in one, or just found your way out of one, *Next!* will help you navigate the exhilarating and occasionally turbulent waters of relationships. Sometimes you'll think you're surfing the perfect wave, and other times you'll think you're drowning—welcome to the cycle of love!

Next! provides you with a blueprint of what to expect from dating all the way through divorce and back again to dating. That's not to say that your marriage won't last; in fact, I offer you tons of advice on how to hold onto a good marriage and keep it exciting. I want every woman to be aware of her relationship options at each stage and to never feel like she is stuck or has to "settle." There is always the next step, the next choice, the next attitude, or the next love interest to keep you moving forward with your romantic life. You never know at which relationship phase you might find yourself, so why not get trained on the whole rotation?

Books on dating end with finding a great catch. Well, what happens after you get engaged? You have to buy a new book for advice about that. *Next!*, on the other hand, will take you through *all* of the relationship stages to prepare you for what lies ahead as well as help you understand what you've left behind. Furthermore, there is an overlapping of skills and attitudes that carry on from one step to the next. For example, it's a good idea to keep the "dating" in marriage by making fun, romantic plans so that the playful part of the relationship stays alive.

Where do you want to go next with your love life? You always have to ask yourself that question and not be afraid to take action. I will help you to overcome your fears and embrace the strength inside of you so that you can make the most of love (and, if you want, make the most love)!

What's in It for You?

If you're like many women whose relationships have left them feeling as motionless as a car that's been sitting in the garage going nowhere, it's time to turn the key in the ignition, grab the steering wheel, and peel out of the driveway. You've got somewhere to get to or get away from!

It's important to know that there are many "someones" out there for everyone, and love starts first and foremost with you. I'll help you write a list of what you're looking for in a relationship in order to keep your singles search focused. I'll cover the do's and don'ts of dating. I'll talk about how to forge a new relationship, evaluate whether it's working, keep a relationship fiery in the bedroom and beyond, make the leap into marriage and children, recognize red flags, move on when all signs point to the door, and recover from a breakup to love another day.

A major part of my relationship philosophy is to just get out there and live. Don't be afraid to make mistakes. Don't get stuck. Always create movement and momentum in your relationships so that they are always going somewhere. When our love lives become stagnant, our happiness levels drop, and we get the sense that we're missing out on a life that could be lived much more fully. Furthermore, when we're unhappy in a relationship, it takes a toll on our health. As a breast-cancer survivor and nutrition-and-fitness enthusiast, I do not take my physical health for granted and neither should you!

With many opportunities to be in stable, fulfilling relationships, no woman needs to resign herself to accepting less than what she wants— whether that means staying with a guy who won't make a marriage commitment, remaining in a marriage where the respect is gone, or buying into the mentality that she's not worthy of love. We deserve love, and can and will find it, not just in one person but in many (should we choose). If you've got a keeper, I'll help you hold onto him through the rough spots. If it's time to release a bad match into the sea of love, I will help you unhook him from your line and wipe the fishy smell from your hands. If you're ready to start from scratch like a fresh cookie for the baking, I'm there for you, too, and will pre-heat the oven. Remember, this book is called *"Next!"* for a reason.

Meet Your Matchmaker

I have been a professional matchmaker since 1986 and have matched over 300 couples who married. I also work as a relationship coach and seminar leader. Driving all of these endeavors is my desire to bring more love into people's lives. I want people to love themselves and others and to gather as much love as they can—from within, from friends, family, romantic partners, children, and pets—while on this wonderful Earth. In my opinion, how much love you've collected along the way is the best way to judge how well you're living.

As far as my own personal relationships are concerned, I've gone to the college of life and graduated with four husbands. Yes, you read that right: four! (Note that the fourth is still in the picture and his nickname is "Lucky.") I am the ultimate recycler. Now, I know learning that I have a herd of ex-husbands will shock some of you and put off others. That's fine, but I will say this: in each case I had real reasons to leave; all of those relationships lasted a significant amount of time (seventeen, six, and ten years); and I come to you with decades of experience—decisions good and bad and insights that only lots of living and loving can provide. Between all of my personal relationships and the relationships I've set in motion through matchmaking or helped through coaching, I am giving Cupid a run for his money.

I celebrate people who have stayed in relationships, and I celebrate people who have left. It's all about doing what's right for you and the other person. By letting someone go, you're not only giving yourself a second chance, but you're also helping him find where he needs to go next.

There is no sense in focusing on the negatives. I believe in squeezing the juice out of those lemons and making the sweetest lemonade your ex-boyfriend will never taste. That's not to say you can't cry or get upset, but too much discouragement brings you down and keeps you there. Whether you're having difficulty dating or a hard time getting over a breakup, you're going to be fine. The lifeboat is there and, lucky you, the captain is 6′3″, blond, rugged, and only has eyes for you! Next!

As you read these words right now, brand-new couples are meeting for the first time in coffee shops and grocery stores around the world. Would you like to be one of them? Or would you like to strengthen the relationship you're presently in?

The world is spinning, and that revolving door constantly stays in motion. Who or what is next for you? What the heck are you waiting for, woman? Let *Next!* get you on your way.

There's Always Someone for Everyone

Not "The One," but Someone

THERE'S SOMEONE OUT THERE FOR EVERYONE. I truly believe that.

You always have to feel in your heart that you will meet a person who is going to love you for who you are. Now I am certainly not saying there is only *one* someone out there for you. I don't believe in the concept of "the one." You're probably thinking, well, evidently you don't, Barbara, since you've had the first "one," and then the next "one," and the next quite a few times.

As my parade of husbands demonstrates, there are a lot of potential matches out there—at least for me. But of course I am not here to promote the concept of multiple marriages or to say that having one husband for life is not a wonderful path, because it is—as long as it's built on mutual respect and devotion. I'm also not here to tell you that you need to get married. What I'm here to do is to help you find and/or keep love, whether it's for the first time or the fifteenth. That's what I do for a living. That's my occupation and personal passion.

Sometimes people get caught up in the mentality that if they were in a long-term relationship that didn't last—whether or not it was a marriage—they don't want to look for love again because they feel that there is not going to be another who can fill that person's shoes. I believe there are a lot of choices out there and that it's up to us to find them.

Why bother with the not-always-easy search? It's all about love.

Love Is All You Need

Love is a feeling and an exalted word. When a romantic partner tells you he loves you, it's like a surround sound of bliss; you're hearing the highest level of appreciation and fulfillment that you can get from another person. Being adored validates who you are and what you bring to the world, whether you're twenty or ninety. To say that about yourself is to say I care for and accept who I am inside and out. Love is the top word; there's nothing higher than this.

It's important to give love back. It's a give-and-take thing. And if you don't have that balance of giving and receiving affection, it creates a lot of doubt within yourself. With no one to share an experience with or to appreciate life with you, you can feel empty. Love is centering, and it is completing.

We often learn from our childhoods how to love and be loved. Maybe a woman has a hard time returning a man's affection because she didn't feel cherished by her parents growing up or she didn't have caring relationships with her siblings. Whatever the cause may be, it's extremely important for people to learn to love (no matter their age) and to improve in their ways of demonstrating it.

There are a lot of people in therapy because of the word "love." They tell their therapists that they don't love themselves, and perhaps they never have. These people might be on antidepressants, overweight, or self-destructive with drugs and alcohol because they feel lonely and unvalued.

If you aren't strong enough, you can allow others to destroy you. If you have had relationships one after another where the guy says, "I just don't love you anymore," you are going to struggle to get back on track. Having someone say that he doesn't love you can be devastating.

We all fall apart when experiencing that kind of conversation. I think that if my husband were to come home and announce that he no longer loved me, the pain of those words would be excruciating. It would mean: I don't appreciate you anymore. I don't see any value in you. I can live the rest of my life without you. I don't need you anymore. You add nothing to my life. You're not a good person. You've done something wrong.

You're not attractive to me. All these things and other crazy thoughts go through your head when hearing those words. That's why you should never say you don't love someone during a breakup.

Even if you feel like you hate the other person because of how he's treated you, saying "I don't love you" does not do either of you any good. It's better to take the high road. Also keep in mind that you never know when you might have a change of heart. I've seen couples go through miserable circumstances when they couldn't stand each other, and then they fell in love again.

In my opinion, **love** is the word that is the most powerful for a woman. We grow up wanting to be adored, and we want people to tell us they love us. We want our parents, our partner, and our children to impart this priceless message. How many people are a mess because they hear their kids say, "I don't love you, Mom. I never have"? Good God, you're going to be reaching for a bottle of Xanax if you're told that!

When you find yourself experiencing the ups and downs that come with a relationship, you might ask: Why do I try so hard? The answer is love. You have to stay true to who you are, and if you are well matched romantically, your partner will bring out the goodness in you and help you shine, and you will do the same for him. It's that radiance of love that makes the endeavor worthwhile.

The Outlook on Being Single

Remember the 1950s—when hula hoops and casseroles were all the rage? Well, so was marriage. In 1950, 78 percent of American adults were married. In 2010, by contrast, the rate was 51 percent. Now let's look at those numbers another way: The population of single (unmarried) adults catapulted from 22 percent in 1950 to 49 percent in 2010. My guess, as we enter 2015, is that the number of singles will continue to rise.

The growth of singlehood and the decline of marriage reflect major changes in our society. People are waiting, on average, much longer before they marry, and many people view the idea of marriage as passé. It's common for people to choose to live together instead of marrying or to cohabitate for a long time before tying the knot. Economic factors play a big role in people's decisions to wait or never say "I do," as well as people's experiences growing up with divorced parents. Many folks are chasing careers and temporary tail. There are all kinds of factors that have contributed to the rise in singles, but that's not what I want to focus on.

Chances are if you're reading this book, you're looking for a *relationship*. It doesn't matter to me if you want that relationship to culminate in marriage or not. You can design whatever works for you.

Secondly, if you're one of those people who feels like an outsider among all your married friends, then please look at the statistics I just cited and realize you've got company. About half of the adults in this country are not married either.

Thirdly, if you've gotten used to not being married or in a relationship, then you might need a shift in attitude before you start dating again. People value their independence; they want to eat dinner when it suits them, watch the shows that they like, and sleep as late as they please on a Sunday. In many ways, people find it easier to be single, to not need to share. Note that I mean *single* here as "not in a relationship" as opposed to the taxpayer status meaning "not married." From here on out, I'm going to use single to signify that someone is not in a committed, exclusive relationship.

If you've gotten comfortable with the single lifestyle, you're going to have to work on adjusting to being part of a couple. It takes effort to balance your life with another person's. Remember that love is give and take, so you've got to be ready for the giving, not just the taking. I think you'll find that the inevitable sacrifices that come with relationships will be worth it, as I don't believe that we're intended to fly solo through life, nor do I think it's a healthy approach.

We're Not Meant to Be Alone

Whether it's evolution or the human origin story from the Bible that you believe in (or something else, but I can't be too politically correct!), both come to the conclusion that humans are not meant to be alone. We are designed to bond intimately with another person in order to procreate and then raise children effectively; we cannot evolve as a species without mating, and it takes two to tango. Or, as the Bible states in Genesis, "God created man in his own image" and told man, "Be fruitful and multiply." Because God saw that "It was not good that the man (Adam) should be alone," God eventually created Eve and put her in the Garden of Eden. Of course, that's when all proverbial hell broke loose, but that's another story.

Now I'm not saying you shouldn't have time alone or some periods of being single. Spending time with your thoughts and pursuing personal interests is vital to your quality of life. It's also not good to jump from one relationship to another without some breaks in between. You don't want to find yourself competing with Dennis Rodman for rebound records. But I don't believe it's healthy to pass the years mostly alone.

Life is all about experiences. Though you can have excellent experiences by yourself, the impact of those adventures is magnified ten-fold when you have someone to share them with. Would you want to go on a hot-air balloon ride alone? You could, but unless you sparked an on-the-spot romance with the balloon operator, it probably wouldn't be as thrilling as going with a partner—popping champagne and gazing at each other as well as the scenery.

When you're in a loving relationship, you also have a strong support structure to rely on. You have someone to talk to about your fears and frustrations and to help you during tough times. Imagine having cancer treatments and then coming home to an empty house. Where would the motivation come from to keep fighting for your survival? A partner helps us in big and small ways to persevere.

When you're alone, you don't have someone to inspire you to take risks or try new endeavors. You stay in a box that is comfortable at first but becomes confining. I believe the world is a great deal bigger and open to possibility when you're sharing it intimately with another person.

I've always thought that the symbol of the heart looks like two bodies coming together. Likewise, I believe that to feel whole in our hearts we have to be partaking of the good life with someone we consider remarkable.

Some people say to me that single women can be happy in the long term without a romantic partner. That's true, in my opinion, but only to a certain extent. Let's say a divorcee has grown children in their twenties and lots of interests, such as volunteering and yoga. She has love coming into her life from many sources, and she's not looking for a man to validate who she is. That's really okay. But it's going to show. It's going to show in her character—in her abruptness and attitude. She's probably not going to be a well woman, because romantic love sustains your health; it's a strong ingredient to our soul that keeps us thriving.

Studies have shown, for instance, that being in love decreases the level of the stress hormone cortisol in our bodies and that married people tend to live longer and have fewer heart attacks, battles with cancer, and bouts with pneumonia than unmarried people.

Let's say you're in your eighties or beyond and single. The idea of getting hot and heavy might make you or your younger relatives gag, but as my mother says, "I don't know a woman alive at any age who wouldn't want a kiss!" Even a kiss on the cheek can give people a romantic charge. A partner you find appealing late in your years could be a man you see two to three nights a week for companionship, someone who wants the best for you, who will hold your hand and make you a strong drink when you need one. And if you can and want to do the horizontal mambo, more power to you!

Love the One You're with: YOU!

Now before you get gaga with the idea of romantic love, let me say that I do not believe for one second that people can be in love with others and yet not love themselves.

Love starts with you: You must take care of yourself and love yourself before you can successfully pair up with another person. Sure, lots of people with poor self-image are in relationships, but what is the quality of those relationships?

For instance, have you ever been with a guy with low self-esteem who drank himself into oblivion every night? You most likely bathed him with attention and affection (until you just couldn't take it anymore) and, try as he might, he couldn't reciprocate in equal measure. That doesn't mean he didn't love you, but because you were a caretaker and he was wallowing in self-loathing, he couldn't be "in the moment" and truly in love with you, and that was devastating. We can't help those who won't help themselves first.

When you aren't happy with yourself, it's hard to let your light shine on another person. As a matchmaker, I've had to tell people seeking my services that matchmaking may not be the right place for them at that point in time. Sometimes they need to seek help elsewhere, whether it's with a nutritionist, therapist, trainer, life coach, or other professional. We're not broken cars; you can't just move some parts around and get people up and running again. We have to work on the parts of ourselves—mental, physical, and emotional—that trouble us.

If you're really insecure about your weight, for instance, or struggling with panic attacks, I suggest you start working on those issues before you try to find a good match. We're all works in progress, and there is no perfect time to find love, but when you are really struggling to love and accept yourself, it's important to address the reasons why. As you start to see progress and an improved self-image, you will be better positioned to kindle a romantic interest.

If you're in a relationship that's floundering, ask yourself if you are loving yourself and doing your best. You may find that you're frustrated with your job or feeling out of shape. Those perceptions and the emotions that come with them might be taking a toll on you and your relationship. Likewise, is your husband or boyfriend down on himself in some way? Is that hurting your relationship? The root of all love begins with the self. We should start there.

But since we're not destined to be alone, once you get yourself to a place of relative comfort and self-acceptance (relative because it's an ongoing process), let's get you back out in the dating scene. Contrary to what some women believe, dating is fun, not a "process," as some grumps refer to it. Pretend you're the star in your own personal version of *Sex and the City*; I'm your wing woman. Now let's get to it!

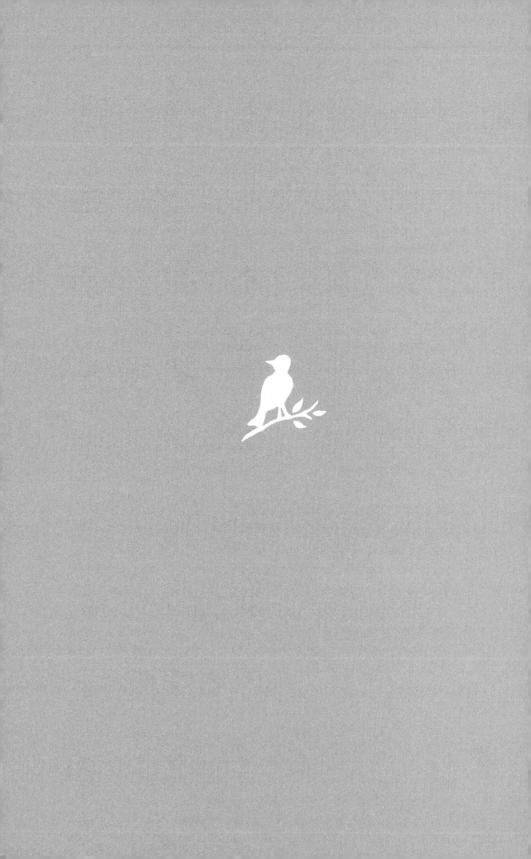

Get Ready for Love

I KNOW A LOT OF WOMEN who have gone to psychics hoping to discover what the romantic future holds. They want to know who awaits them or if the relationships they're in will last. Women are natural worriers. We should be natural warriors, but we often fret about everything imaginable, including our love lives. We're driven by hope and want answers. Women want to be told that things will get better, that we'll be safe, that life will have positive outcomes.

I can't look into a crystal ball to see whether you'll receive more marriage proposals than Elizabeth Taylor, but I can reveal this about your future: if you're single and want love, you will find it! As I'll discuss in this chapter, it's all about belief in yourself and preparation.

Face Fear

A lot of people are afraid of dating and becoming involved in new relationships. Whether it's worry about picking the wrong person, anxiety about STDs, rejection, introducing a new partner to their children, or getting physical too quickly, single people often let these fears keep them on the sidelines.

Fear is the biggest obstacle to any endeavor. Once you allow it to enter your life, it's like hitting the brakes. You stop the possibility of anything good happening to you.

There are risks with dating, as there are with anything in life. Therefore it's natural to be a little nervous. You need to take precautions, as I'll discuss in chapter five, but you also need to get out there and make things happen. Love is not going to strike you when you're sitting alone in your one-bedroom apartment on a Friday night eating ice cream.

Love is the ultimate goal, and to reach it you're going to have to get back on the proverbial horse and ride. It starts with preparation.

Prepare for a Relationship

You have to put yourself in a positive headspace to be able to open up to the idea of dating. Part of that process is making sure you feel good about who you are and the image you present to the world. You might need a simple redo to pluck you out of your doom and gloom, like a different haircut or new way of applying cosmetics—or perhaps have a professional makeover. Celebrate yourself with a fresh start. Go shopping for an outfit you might wear on a date, like an elegant dress or trendy jeans and a beautiful sweater. Get excited. Refresh yourself. Return to an exercise routine, whether just going on walks with a girlfriend or sweating it out at the gym. Or take that pottery workshop you've been eyeing.

The point is to slowly get some of your energy back. Maybe you haven't noticed, but you've probably been what I call flat-lined: stuck in the muck of life, a blah, uninspired place that you need to leave behind.

After making yourself feel prettier and recharged, do the same with your home. Eventually this new person is going to see where you live. Maybe you need to get rid of clutter or pull up weeds in the backyard. Home improvement in this sense could be as simple as buying fresh flowers and displaying them on the dining room table. If you're the kind of girl who has everything you own in the backseat of your car, including last week's coffee cups, clean out your car.

Spruce up items a new person might use when going on a date with you, such as sports equipment or a picnic basket. If you have a dog, get him groomed. Get ready for the fact that you are going to find love. Don't think: Why would I do all this? This is a waste of time. You're doing this because you are going to find a connection that will lead to a wonderful relationship, so you might as well fix up yourself and your house, car, and golf clubs the way you want to.

If you're a single mom and your children haven't been minding you, start working with your kids. Let them know that mom is going to start dating and is going to find love. They might give you a hard time, but you need to start preparing them. Preparation on every level is extremely important.

Thirdly, get support. The best way to do that is to open your mouth and start telling people, "I'm thinking about dating." Your friends and family members or whoever you turn to for encouragement will say, "That's terrific! Do you want to join my coed soccer team?" Or, "My coworker's brother, who is super hot, is recently single. I'm going to introduce you!"

The worst thing you can do is to be quiet about your plans. Think of it this way: If you want a job in advertising, would it be a better strategy to be silent about it or to tell many people? The answer is obvious. From talking to people, you might find out that your friend's cousin runs an advertising firm that's hiring.

You're not going to execute anything if it's only in your thoughts. Share it. Say it aloud. If you're in therapy, tell your therapist you plan on dating. Even talk to yourself in the mirror. "Mirror, mirror on the wall, I'm going to find a magnificent relationship for myself this year. It's going to happen." There. You said it. Your mind accepted it. And you're going to do the work needed to find this person.

On the flipside, if you have doubt—"I don't know if I can do this. I don't think I can find anyone"—then you're right. It's not going to happen. You just doubted it. Your mind heard it. And you're done. The brain is very powerful. I always say the subconscious can't take a joke, so be careful what you tell it. You might have a lot of negative feelings about dating: all men are jerks, or every guy I meet has had major problems. You can't talk to yourself that way. You need to be open and receiving, and you have to work through your fears verbally.

I know this from being a cancer survivor. After having a sample tissue from my left breast removed, I told the doctor as I was being wheeled out of surgery, "My breast tissue is going to be perfect. There's going to be no cancer in it." He looked at me and said, "We'll know in about ten days." I said, "No, I'm telling you right now. It's going to be healthy." I went home and every night I visualized my body being cancer-free. Sure enough, days later I got a call that confirmed it. I'm not saying that would work every time, but I believe if you follow your heart and mind and make them connect, there are many possibilities.

I had a client who was a good-looking guy in his late 30s, but the right side of his face was paralyzed. He was born that way. I remember his deflated energy when he came in my office the first time. He started off by apologizing for the way he looked. I said, "Stop this, Sean. We're going to find a woman who will love you for who you are." He was a physical therapist and talented artist. We talked for two and a half hours, and I realized he had a marvelously kind manner that would make someone very happy. I instilled him with hope for a match and made him feel good about himself and his passions. He told me he didn't care what the woman looked like as long as she didn't care what he looked like.

I set out searching. Now, I'll be honest. It was not easy to find a match for him. After one year, I found the perfect girl. Beverly was always fighting her weight and was a sassy, bossy kind of girl. She didn't see anything wrong with Sean and thought he was extremely handsome and charming. He always wanted to please her and thought she was wonderful; Beverly had never felt as good about herself as she did with Sean. It didn't matter that she needed to lose twenty pounds. It worked, and they are adorable together. They got married and now have three children! Like Sean, you can get rid of the negativity and the doubt and visualize love coming your way, and it will.

Create Some Room

To be ready for a relationship, you've got to make room. If you cram your schedule with church groups, tennis lessons, ladies nights, volunteering at an animal shelter, raising children, and working full time, where do you envision a guy stepping in?

Assess how you're living your life to see whether there is space for a man. How is he going to fit into your day-to-day existence as it stands now? Some single women keep their lives stuffed to the point that they're essentially blocking Mr. Right's way. It could be low self-esteem, a fear of sex, a fear of change, or any number of reasons why women—intentionally or not—make it difficult for men to even find time to schedule a date with them.

A client named David called me recently to say, "I really liked Sarah, but she doesn't have any time for me. I asked her out again and she said she couldn't see me for two weeks." He explained that her daughters were visiting, she had a class to take, Bible study three nights a week, and several other "obligations." I called Sarah and asked, "Did you like David?" She said, "Oh gosh, he's great. We had a wonderful date; it lasted six hours."

I can't stand it when women pull the I'm-too-busy card! I raised my voice and asked, "Then why is it that he wants to take you out, but you can't see him for two weeks?" She starts, "Well, Barbara . . ." I'm thinking, well, nothing. I let her rattle off her excuses and then cut to the quick. "I thoroughly understand your position, Sarah, but here's my situation. I'm representing David, and I'm not going to let him sit out there for two weeks to wait to go out with you again. I've got two other women who I'm going to set him up with while you figure it out. If he likes them, that's too bad. If he doesn't, you're lucky."

Of course she says, "Well, wait a minute." Women like Sarah start backpedaling and suddenly, miracle upon miracle, they come up with time for the guy. I've needed to have many conversations like that in my matchmaking career. Ladies, if you want to find love, don't make your schedule like a maze where the guy has to run down all kinds of dead ends to eventually find that little piece of cheese. Unless the guy is one desperate, starving mouse, he's just not going to try that hard.

When I'm interviewing potential matchmaking clients, I have to climb into their lives and take a look around to ensure that I feel comfortable setting them up. I remember one woman named Debbie who sought my services. When I interviewed her, I found out she had five cats and two dogs. Her three young children (all under five years old) were not all from the same father, which made her custody schedule complicated. Debbie worked nights and had every other weekend free.

You know how people talk in a hysterical whisper when they're stressed out? Well, that was Debbie. In her frazzled manner, she looked like a hissing cat whose hair stands on end. Naturally, I'm sitting there thinking: How is this going to work? Just finding a guy who wants to be around that many animals is a real challenge, never mind everything else she has going on. I had this picture in my head of a guy showing up at the front door, and these cats would be running up the staircase and jumping from the chandelier onto his shoulders. And then he would sprint back to his car and drive away as fast as he could.

I expressed my doubts to her, and in her strange, whispering way, she practically screamed at me, "But I'm a really good match!" I said, "Debbie, I bet you are, but I'm trying to envision this." In matchmaking it's a waste of everybody's time (including mine) when a person is not ready to date. I could set someone up over and over again, but it's never going to work if that person's life is a mess. I told Debbie that if she wanted to work with me, she first had to reinvent how she was living her life. I gave her a lot of suggestions, including changing her work schedule and giving away the kittens; her cat had recently had a litter that she was thinking of keeping because she was having a hard time finding homes for them.

Sorry, PETA, but I don't know many men who love cats. Maybe it's because cats can't be controlled, and men don't like anything they can't control to some degree. That's not to say that you shouldn't have a cat if you want one, but you don't want to end up a crazy spinster cat lady with nine cats instead of a husband.

To her credit, Debbie made major changes. She pursued a different occupation and landed a day job with weekends free. She gave away the kittens and signed up for the babysitting service I recommended for her children. Debbie also touched up her hair with a new cut and colored the early gray. She looked and acted much happier.

In a funny twist, I set her up with a dog breeder who was more of an animal lover than she was. One day he showed up in my office covered in dog hair with a big grin on his face. I thought to myself, I know just the person for you! He didn't have or want any children of his own, but he was happy to take on hers. It worked out very well. He was an upbeat, carefree type, which allowed her to roll parts of her lifestyle over into his because nothing seemed to bother him. But if Debbie hadn't made some big changes, she would have been too much to handle, even for Mr. Mellow. They got married and are one large, jolly family brimming over with kids and puppies and cat fur.

Leave the Ex Behind

Occasionally I don't pick up the signal that a woman isn't ready to start dating, and I set her up with someone. The next day I get a call from the guy she went out with that starts with statements like, "Barbara, this is not going to work. All she did was go on and on about her ex-husband. I think she's still in love with him." The only time you should ramble on about an ex during a date is if you're hoping the guy will never call you again.

As we discussed in the previous chapter, there are times when women think they're ready to be in a relationship, but they really are not. Whether it's working on loving yourself first or making sure you're over your ex, there's a certain amount of mental shifting that needs to go on before your date's assured that you're not mental.

The first priority after a breakup is to bring life back into yourself. You don't need someone else's life to take on. It can be hard to be alone, especially if you've been with a partner for a number of years, but you have to go through the process. Otherwise, you'll be a dating disaster. Trust me. It's far better to shed those tears over the phone with a friend than on the sleeve of your first date. Get some exercise, reach out to friends and family, pursue your passions, stay busy, and recreate your joie de vivre.

Even if the breakup was amicable, you've still been hurt. You need time to adapt to change and to learn to be on your own again. After a relationship ends, it's important to reconnect with who you are, a person separate from the man who was in your life.

I know a woman who proceeded to tell a man on their first date that she still thought of herself as an extension of her husband, even though her husband had been dead for five years. She didn't perceive herself as anything other than Mrs. So and So. While I sympathize with her discomfort, this is a big dating and life mistake. You must have a strong personal identity apart from your relationship identity. Without confidence in who you are, finding your way (never mind a match) will be very difficult. From a dating perspective, guys don't want to be with a woman who can't be alone and who doesn't know herself beyond the bounds of the relationship.

After a relationship loss—whether it's due to death, divorce, or a breakup—you have to figure out what your needs are and what it's going to take to get strong mentally and physically. I know women who became almost anorexic after a relationship went sideways. They fell apart, dropped twenty pounds, and went on antidepressants. They had to work to get back to a healthy balance of eating right, feeling optimistic, and believing in their worth before they could start dating again. Make sure you, too, are healed and ready before you even think of accepting a date.

Don't take with you into the next relationship all of your memories of what it was like to be with your ex. Identify with those experiences. Learn from them. But don't carry them over; you want a new beginning, not a sloppy remake.

I'll talk about breakups more in future chapters, but for now, ask yourself if you're mostly over your ex. Do you think the relationship ended for good reasons and that you are ready to move on? If the answer is "yes," great. If it's "no" or "I'm not sure" or "I hope we get back together," then wait until you're truly prepared before dating again.

All right, ladies, I hope you've started to face your fears about dating and to make plans for improving yourself and your environment. Remember to unclutter your life so that Mr. Right doesn't sprain his ankle on the way in. And be positive! Doom and gloom is not an aphrodisiac and will never be prescribed as a love cure. So look in the mirror at that gorgeous head of hair wrapped in a towel and skin covered in face cream and say, "Love is on the way, good-looking." Be sure to seal the pep talk with a smile and a victory dance.

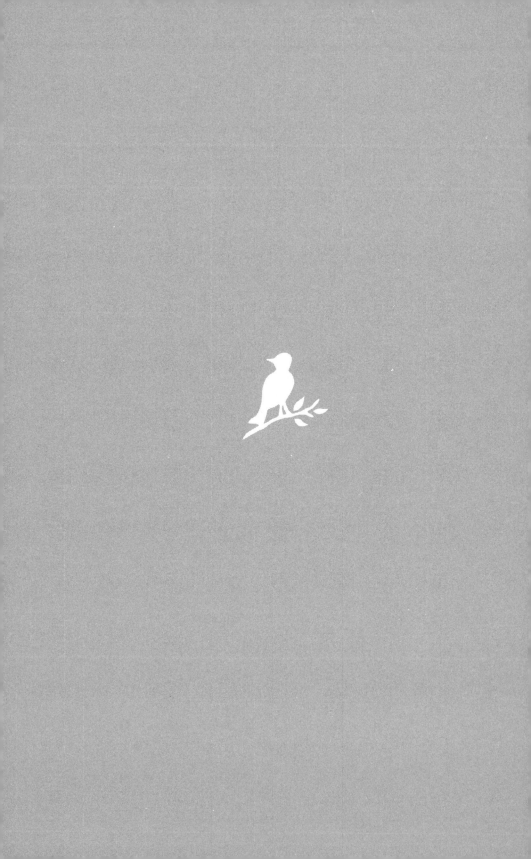

The List:
Creating Your Dream Match

PREPARATION IS VERY IMPORTANT because you could meet the right guy right away but blow your chances by not being ready for a relationship. It's like looking for a house. The first one the realtor shows you might be amazing. You think it's everything you want, but you hold off on making an offer because it's the first house you've seen. Meanwhile, someone else scoops it, and you find yourself regretting your failure to act.

Timing is responsible for many of our life events. Within a week a guy could meet two women he really likes. The one who is ready for a relationship is probably going to be the one he ends up with. Being ready, as we discussed last chapter, is making room, having time, being over your ex, getting into an encouraging headspace, and working on a better you.

Part of the preparation process also involves knowing what you're looking for in a partner, which brings us to "the list."

What You Reflect and Attract

When I have new matchmaking clients, I ask them to describe their dream man or woman. As they're talking, I write down their wished for characteristics. People tend to start with physical appearance and then move on to personality traits and lifestyle. Sometimes they get so carried away that I have to ask them to whittle down their list, but that's another story that I'll get to momentarily.

At the end of this chapter I am going to ask you to write your own Dream Match List, so read carefully and start thinking about what you're looking for in Mr. Right. However, keep in mind that it's not a "Dream Match" as in a delusional fantasy (think Leonardo DiCaprio) but an attainable, yet cherished ideal.

When I ask clients to tell me their list, in my mind I want to visualize what they seek in a partner, because I believe that two individuals in a relationship mirror each other. First of all, people usually search for a partner with a similar level of physical attractiveness. The Angelina Jolies find the Brad Pitts. Style also comes into play: the hipster wearing skinny jeans skips over the man in a tailored suit to go for the guy sporting Buddy Holly glasses and an ironic t-shirt. Of course I am speaking in generalities, and there are many exceptions. What's important is that I hear what my clients say they are looking for in another person's appearance because it tells me to a certain extent how they see themselves.

Secondly, the people we draw toward us usually reflect the way that we're living our lives at that particular snapshot in time. The guy who drives a Porsche and climbs corporate America's ladders of success is probably going to seek another ambitious, image-driven person, while the young woman going through a rebellious phase might match up with an equally unruly guy or perhaps search for someone to straighten her out. These of-the-moment tendencies can lead to long-term incompatibility. The guy with the Porsche, for example, could find that his hot blonde really just liked him for his money and left him in the breakdown lane when he lost his job. The young woman could discover that the guy with the tattoos and piercings who nursed her through a drug addiction when she was nineteen is not the guy she wants to play tennis with when she's forty.

Part of the reason I advise people to start dealing with their personal struggles before they get into relationships is because when the problems that initially brought a couple together (dependence on drugs, financial troubles, low self-esteem, and so forth) are removed, or a life situation changes drastically, sometimes there's no place left for the two people to go. One partner grows this way; the other grows that way, and both find that there's no long-term value in the relationship.

When it comes time for you to draft your list of what you're attempting to find in a partner, ask yourself what that list is saying about how you perceive yourself. Adjust the list and the way you're living if you think you're limiting your horizons.

Must-Haves, Nice-to-Haves, and Deal Breakers

What is it that you definitely want in a guy? What would be nice to have but not absolutely necessary? What would you certainly not put up with?

Let's say you're physically active and love to exercise, so couch potatoes need not apply. Maybe your guy has to love children and want to have them. Perhaps you seek someone who is respectful, warm-hearted, has an occupation, doesn't drink too much, and is self-supporting (pays his bills without bumming money off you). Maybe you didn't finish college and you're okay with him not having a degree as long as he has a purpose and is focused. Ideally you'd like the guy to be a frequent beach-goer because hanging out at the shore is one of your favorite weekend activities. Does he have to be taller than you? Yes?

Okay, as your matchmaker, I'll be on the lookout for a man who exercises, wants to have a baby, is financially solid, taller than you, kind, and hopefully has a college degree and enjoys rays and days at the beach. If you add any additional requirements beyond that, you might have to pay me more. I wish it worked that way, as I'd make a lot more money!

I've had female clients say to me, "He needs to be 6′2″ or taller with broad shoulders and be in great shape. He can't be going bald. He has to have thick hair, come from a wealthy family, drive a BMW, Mercedes, or Lexus, and live in Del Mar or Solana Beach. (He can't be inland because I don't want to drive.) He must own his own home and make a six-figure salary. He also has to be willing to wear suits and know designer clothing." I'll look across the table at the woman and think, all righty then. Maybe if you were a Cameron Diaz we could be describing this guy, but I'm just not seeing it. I'll return to the divas a little later in this chapter.

Now, if you're young, very attractive, make a sizable income, are well educated, and have other attributes that make you a ten, then you can rattle off what you want and expect to find it. Most of the time though, the longer the list, the longer you're going to be single.

That's why when writing your list, you need to decide what is an absolute must, what is a wish, and what is a deal breaker. For instance, using the example of the hypothetical woman who led off this section, her must-haves are a man who is respectful, has a career, financially supports himself, exercises, and is kind. Having a college degree and being a beach-lover are on her wish list. The deal breakers would be a guy not wanting kids, drinking too much, and being shorter than her. On your list I suggest having no more than five must-haves, five wishes, and five deal breakers.

When you're coming up with your list, keep in mind that lifestyle is the number-one thing that makes or breaks a relationship, not height or eye color or six-pack abs turning to flab. I always ask clients the question: What is your typical Sunday like? If you're a girl who paints landscapes and enjoys bird watching, you're not going to want the guy who paints his face silver and black and tailgates at Raiders games.

Search for someone who enjoys at least a few of the activities that you do. At the same time, a relationship can be like a semester in college that exposes you to new ideas and practices. You want a partner who brings knowledge and value into your life and who brings you out of your box. If a person is just like you, it will get boring. But if the guy is not enough like you, there will be tension. So, when I'm matching I look for commonalities between lists, but I also look for a little zest—hobbies and interests that can spice up both people's lives.

If the guy has to be an avid biker because you spend at least one day a weekend bombing around on two wheels, put it on the must-have list. If it's not absolutely necessary, yet it is important to you, put it on the wish list. But be open to the possibility that you could introduce him to biking and he could get you into, let's say, photography.

Dancing shows up often on women's wish lists. Women will say to me, "I'd love for him to know how to dance or be willing to learn." Dancing represents a letting go; it's fun and festive. Women don't want the guy who, when trying to protect his ego, just sits at the table gulping down his drink. Females who enjoy dancing get resentful when they're stuck in their chairs tapping their toes because their guys won't get up and join them on the dance floor. Take note, male readers, and learn how to shake that thing! No, not that thing!

Temperament is very important to consider when you're writing your list. You need to really think about the character traits that work best for you. Is your Mr. Right easygoing? Intellectual? Talkative? A sense of humor is good to have, as well as confidence that doesn't border on narcissism.

Whatever you do, don't let your list go to hell because the guy is good-looking. Attraction is often a detour from your list. His breathtaking blue eyes and muscular arms will lose their appeal when he chooses to surf every day instead of work. You can be very physically attracted to a man who is not a good fit for you now and never will be.

Let's face it: when people are young, they're very driven by looks. That's fine, twentysomethings, but make sure there's substance behind his gorgeous exterior. Some say that as you get up there in age, you're just looking for a warm body and hoping he's got all his marbles. In my opinion, even if you're 95, you should make sure he meets your minimum list requirements. Can still chew his own food? Check. Is willing to stroll around the block, even if it's in a wheelchair? Check.

I never allow my clients to see photos of their matches before the first date. Sometimes a picture makes people appear better than they really are, and sometimes it makes them appear worse. Also, you can't experience an individual's essence through a photo as well as you can in person. That's why I tell my clients to trust me and go see for themselves.

Now, there should also be deal breakers on your list in addition to the must-haves and nice-to-haves. Everyone's deal breakers are different, whether they have to do with children, religion, finances, or something else.

Recently I found a girl, Karen, who I thought was going to be perfect for an eye doctor I was representing. She's stunningly beautiful, 54 years old, 5′11″, and has a nice personality. We met for coffee, and Karen's list, as well as her answers to my questions, seemed like a terrific fit for Tom. During the hour-and-a-half interview, I was itching to call him with the good news. At the café I started to gather my things to go, thinking we were finished, when suddenly Karen said, "I have to tell you the two most important things that have to be in my life with a partner."

I picked up my pen again. Guess what we didn't cover? Drinking and religion. She's in Alcoholics Anonymous and prefers that the guy not drink. Karen also goes to church four days a week and wants a religious partner. Wha wha. I almost broke the pen. Tom has a wine cellar and is an atheist. Religion is the hardest list item for me to work around, much more than drinking or even politics. Like Karen, if you have religious deal breakers, then start there. Target people who fit your religious requirements *first*.

Let Experience Shape Your List

I learned from my own relationships what needed to be on my list. For example, after divorcing my husband who had been an NFL football player, I decided I wanted someone who had been in a profession that he loved for over ten years. Luke was retired from football when we got married, and over the course of our relationship, he never found another career that he was passionate about. It's interesting to note that Luke became a handyman with a thriving business after we split up, which has given him great professional joy. Sometimes the people we love can't find their identity with us, which is why breakups can be blessings in disguise. At the time of our divorce, I had a grown daughter, as well as grandchildren, so I wanted someone who also had grown children and who could relate to what that entailed.

After Luke and I split up, I subscribed to *Travel & Leisure* magazine and envisioned embarking on fabulous trips. I put that desire out there in my mind as I started to date again. I had an interest in golf but couldn't afford golf clubs at that time (the divorce wiped me clean), but I found cheap ways to rent clubs and play. And then I met Robert, who is now my husband. He is a certified public accountant who loves his work. He has grown children and young grandchildren and is a dedicated family man who cares for his quadriplegic brother. Robert enjoys traveling and golf. He had the list items I was looking for, and vice versa, which made us compatible. The rest, as they say, is history.

Take your breakups and spread them on the coffee table in front of you. What do they reveal? What are they teaching you to look for, moving forward? Use your experiences—good and bad—to create your list.

Right now I have a very wealthy client named Scott who has been difficult to match up. Part of the problem is that for the past six months Scott was searching for a knockout without being one himself. And then one day it dawned on him. He told me that neither of his ex-wives were nurturing. Scott said their attitude was like they were doing him a favor by being with him. As a result, he decided to change his requirements. The woman doesn't have to be smoking hot. He just wants someone who is real and who will celebrate him for who he is. We all deserve to find a partner who will make us a priority and cherish us, but that only happens when we are being real ourselves.

Don't Be Over the Top (The Diva Complex)

When Robert and I got married, I was crazy busy with work. He helped me scale back my matchmaking business in a way that allowed me to be profitable but have free time. That's definitely a perk to sharing your life with an accountant—he can track my finances all the way down to a water bill. When Robert asked me what I'd like to change about my business, I said, "I am really tired of working with these women who come to me with unrealistic expectations." He responded, "Well, why don't you just work with men?"

After years and years of dealing with women who had over-the-top ideas of what the guy should look like and what kind of money he should make, I decided in 2003 to start working almost exclusively with men. (Occasionally I'll take a female client if she's realistic.) With men as my clients, I can be in charge of the women. I used to get these demanding females who wanted me to match them with guys who stood 6′2″ or taller with dark hair, green eyes, and muscular builds who made $150,000 to $200,000 a year. If the woman made a lot of money, I understood her desire for a man with a similar income, but often the fantasy man's income was a huge step up from hers. And it was always the 5′2″ girl who had to have the giant. Why? They needed to feel little. Hello, 5′2″, you're already little. Check yourself out in the mirror. A guy who is 5′10″ is not going to make you feel little?

These high-maintenance women would say things like: He can't be a renter. He can't have children. He must ski. I have to be able run every day. I used to listen until I just couldn't stand it anymore. With the really ridiculous ones I'd say, "I'll be back in fifteen minutes and when I return, I want to see this list cut in half." Some of them, though, just could not be whipped into shape.

Since launching my business, I have been brought to small claims court once. A female client, Plain Jane, wanted her money back because she said I didn't match her up with anyone suitable. Even though my contract says I guarantee three introductions, I set her up with six really great guys. Plain Jane didn't think any of them were good-looking enough. She was ten pounds overweight and not very attractive, yet she thought the guy needed to have the sex appeal of Ryan Gosling. In court, I read aloud her list. I also approached the bench and showed the judge the files and pictures of the guys I matched her with. He said, "You've got to be joking. What did you find wrong with any of these men?" Plain Jane argued that they weren't attractive enough. The judge hit the gavel to the desk and declared the case closed with me as the winner.

When men are paying me to match them, they are ready to go. They don't want to be single, and they are serious about finding someone. Women often tell me they're ready for a relationship, but in actuality they're not. They won't make the time or the effort or be realistic in their expectations. In business, you sell time. An hour with a contractor or chiropractor will cost you a certain amount of money. In a relationship, you are selling your time as well, so neither party appreciates it when the other wastes that precious, ticking resource.

That's not to say that I don't get male clients who frustrate me. I remember one guy kept insisting that I match him with a brunette with light eyes. Finally I said to him, "Are you telling me that you can't get a hard-on if she has brown eyes? Go get her colored contacts and play sex games." I mean, seriously, get over it. I can't snap my fingers and produce the "perfect" woman or man. We aren't images in a catalog and if you don't want to be single, you're going to have to learn the difference between fantasy and reality.

Check in Your Own Baggage

My son-in-law's mother did not welcome my daughter, Leisa, into the fold. At the time of their engagement, Leisa's daughter (my granddaughter), Morgan, was six years old. This wasn't what Mark's mother envisioned for her oldest child, who had been single until he was forty, owned three properties, and was an accomplished businessman. She didn't like the "baggage" that Leisa carried.

Baggage. I hate that word. Is character baggage? Is experience baggage? You can't have a life before your current relationship? You can't have children, pets, or a former spouse?

I've had clients say they want someone with no baggage because they themselves are homeowners with no kids, no pets, and no debts. I remember saying to one particularly smug woman who wanted a baggage-free match, "But you do have baggage." She was shocked and said, "I don't understand—I just presented my case." I thought, you are a case, but I explained to her that because she was fearful of losing control, she kept hitting the brakes and making it impossible for a man to find a way into her life. There was a reason why she was still single and seeking my services. Some people find themselves to be so exceptional and disciplined in their quest for perfection that they never take a chance on anything. As a result, they don't allow an opening for a relationship to flourish.

In my opinion, a lifetime of taking chances is better than a lifetime of playing it safe. Duh! Obviously that's my standpoint; look at the way I've lived my life. I believe nothing ventured, nothing gained, and that people who are willing to take risks are often very successful. But regardless of whether you've put yourself out there or reined yourself in, and regardless of whether you've been married multiple times or single until you were fifty, the key is to be aware of why you made the choices you did and how they've impacted your life. All choices have their ups and downs, and we all have reasons for making our decisions. Those decisions shape us and our character. Each experience is a learning process, and we have to present our lives in the positive. Don't get stuck on regret and what-ifs!

Women's voices will drop when they say, "I'm a single mom." No, be proud of that. You have a family now, and you made the best judgment that you could at the time. You were willing to take a gamble, regardless of whether it worked out. When we say, "I do," we all hope for happily ever after. Sometimes we don't pay attention to the red flags waving in front of our faces. Other times, however, we can be totally blindsided by what meets us in the future. For instance, I never would have guessed that my first husband would end up making extremely bad choices that spiraled out of control and were destructive to himself and me and, ultimately, to our marriage. One of my goals in writing this book is to give people the confidence to take the lessons they learned from their experiences and to move forward toward love.

I recently met an attractive forty-three-year-old woman named Amanda at a party where I was looking for matches. Amanda told me about how her husband's business had collapsed; they filed for bankruptcy and lost the 7,000-square-foot house, the Bentley, and other luxuries. They divorced. When I met her, Amanda had four children under twelve years old; she was renting a small place, and working in a clothing store. Her self-esteem was terrible. She said, "Obviously you shouldn't even consider me as a possible match for your clients."

When she continued to wallow in her sob story, I said, "Stop this right now. Tell me about your children." They are the true jewels, not the Bentley and the other lavish goods. I told Amanda to reframe her thoughts and to look for a man who will make her whole with her family. She needed to have a list of strengths, not a running tally of personal disasters.

I told her, "You can find a guy who believes you're everything he's been looking for." She asked, "Do you really think that?" I said, "Absolutely." Later, I ran into a former client of mine and told him about Amanda. He didn't want to have any children of his own, but he had always wanted to have the experience of raising kids. I set them up, and they really liked each other and have been dating for the past several months.

On the other end of the spectrum, the people who have never married or had children can be very rigid. Some have a picture-perfect image of how they see their future unfolding, but life is rarely like a fairytale. I had one client named Rebecca who said she wouldn't date anyone with children. As I always do when people tell me their lists, I write everything down and try to find what the clients want (assuming their lists are fairly reasonable). However, if I find a potential match who meets many, but not all, of their requirements, I ask clients to trust me that I know what I'm doing and to give something a chance—even if it's something they think they would never tolerate. In this case it was children.

I called Rebecca and said, "The bad news is that Jimmy has a child." She said, "Oh, no, Barbara, I don't want to go out with anyone who has kids!" I said, "All right, just hear me out. Let me tell you about Jimmy and see if you're open to going out with him." I explained that Jimmy's wife had died in a horrible car accident a few years ago. He was raising his son, who is adorable, well mannered, and in kindergarten, by himself, and Jimmy was willing to have another child. I told her that the boy was a beautiful child, not "baggage," and that he would open up her heart and teach her about love. Rebecca hesitantly agreed to give it a chance. Jimmy was the first man I introduced her to, and they got married within a year's time.

Keep the Trophies in Sports

Regarding the dream list, I'd like to give you this last piece of advice: Don't fantasize about marrying a guy with a lot of money who will take care of all your worldly needs as you just sit there and look pretty. Because guess what? Pretty doesn't last very long. We're talking fifteen to twenty years and then it's Botox, hair extensions, and five days a week at the gym.

Being a "trophy wife" comes with a price. You will lose your power to a guy who tells you what to do and how to look. You are much better off having an equitable relationship with a partner who is not only a lover, but also a best friend. Marrying for money can be a disaster. Really, I know very few cases where it has worked out. We all want to be in control over our lives; we don't want to be Stepford wives, allowing the guy to call all the shots while we look sexy and stay out of the way.

Some of you ideally don't want to work. That's fine, but most guys are going to want to see that you aren't just into them for their money. Men like women who have a passion that gives purpose to the woman's life, whether it's a job, volunteering, or a hobby. Women are never going to win by coming from a needy place, because men prefer strong women who can think and act for themselves.

A friend of mine, a hairstylist, once said to me, "I can't work anymore. I've got to find a guy who's got his life together and can support me." I said, "Well, what are you going to give him? What do you bring to the table?" She didn't have an answer. You can't go into dating with the idea that a man is going to get you away from it all—that he's going to save you. You've designed a life for yourself and you need to take responsibility for it—good, bad, and ugly. You have to be willing to work to improve the areas of your life that are unsatisfying, whether it's your job, your relationship with your parents, or your health. Relationships are not one-sided. You don't get to receive without giving, so make sure that you're bringing a list of desirable characteristics to the partnership.

Before you move on to chapter four about finding Mr. Right, sit down right now with a pencil in hand and write your Dream Match List! Please turn to page 192 to get started, where you'll find space for your must-have, would-like-to-have, and won't-have requirements. This is very important! I can't send you out into the singles scene if you're clueless about what you're looking for, because you'll be wasting his time and yours and repeating your previous mistakes. Love is out there. It's a few pick-up tips away. The question is: Are you prepared to find it?

Picking Out and Picking Up Mr. Right

You've got your list in hand and are ready to go. Mr. Right is out there somewhere. But this is the part where many women have trouble. They just daydream. I'm here to tell you that Mr. Right is not going to come to you through your front door, your television, or your romance novel, so you need to get out there, find him, and talk to him. Where is he? How can you get his attention without being obnoxious or flashing your hooters? Read on.

Finding Mr. Right in His Natural Habitat

I believe you should hold off on using online dating and instead try to make real-world connections. The best way to meet someone is through your social network: friends, family members, acquaintances, colleagues, and groups you're affiliated with. By groups, I mean anything from the Young Scandinavians Club to recreational soccer. Between everyone you know and everything you do, you should have a vast network. If you don't, develop it.

Often when I talk to women who are having a hard time meeting guys, it's largely because they don't go out or do much. Expanding your network by getting more involved in activities will not only improve your quality of life. It will also provide more chances to rub elbows with Mr. Right or with a person who knows Mr. Right. Spread the word through your network that you're single and looking to meet someone. This is a great way to get introduced to a guy who comes labeled as a catch. The business world is all about networking. To a large extent, dating is, too.

Get out of the house and socialize. People are attracted to others who are fun and active. When you spend all of your free time watching television, what are you going to have to talk about? What is going to be interesting about you? If you think your lifestyle is boring or you've gotten lazy or uninspired, think of ways to bring excitement into your schedule. Try a meditation class; join an outdoor meet-up group; become a member of your local rotary club. Take part in life. Play. Explore. Interact. Whatever you like or are curious about, do it. Join singles groups that go hiking, bowling, or wine tasting. There are so many possibilities for expanding your social circles. I know several women who have started to run, for instance, because they've noticed how many guys are training for marathons and 5Ks. Getting in shape while hoping Mr. Right will find you cute in lycra is a win-win.

Sometimes when I seek new clients, I go to macho action movies, where I find many single men. I love it when the lights come on because it's like shooting fish in a barrel. I'll ask an attractive man what he thought about the film and then say, "Did your wife not want to watch this movie?" If he says he isn't married, then I tell him I'm a professional matchmaker and explain what I do. If he seems even remotely interested, I give him my card. I've picked up a lot of clients that way, and had I been single I could have picked up dates instead!

For those of you on a tight budget, finding guys does not need to be expensive. It can be part of your daily routine. When I'm looking for matches, for example, I head over to Whole Foods on Sunday between 4 and 7 p.m. Why? Because many single people go grocery shopping at that time. I also stroll through open farmers markets, go to Starbucks, and hang out at fitness clubs. You can volunteer, attend free events, and join free groups.

Be patient. Your quilting class ("stitch and bitch") might not be the best place to meet men, but let's say you make a new female friend there. When you hang out with her, she tells you about a single guy she knows from volunteering for an environmental nonprofit. She invites you to a beach cleanup. You meet him, and he's cute and starts talking to you. By the end of the day he's asked you out. Or, you do the beach cleanup, meet him, and don't particularly connect, but you have a great day doing environmental work and enjoying the company of the people involved. You start to socialize with a few of them, who regularly go to happy hour on Thursday nights. One Thursday night, in walks (insert your dream man here).

The point I'm trying to make is that life happens when you are actively engaged with it, and sometimes the unintended ripple effect of doing one thing, which leads to another, and then to another, is how people meet their mates. It's going to be very difficult to start a relationship if you're a hermit or a couch potato. Shy people can partake of the world around them, too. Shyness doesn't block the way to a gallery opening or a spin class at the gym, though shy people are going to have to work on their vibe (more on that to follow).

If you haven't already noticed, I'm big on verbalization. As you're making the rounds and keeping your eyes peeled for eligible bachelors, I want you to announce five times a day that you're single and looking to meet someone.

Online Dating as a Last Resort

As a matchmaker, I check out people's backgrounds. In many cases, I visit them in their offices or homes, where I look for any heads in the freezer. It's always a relief when I only find popsicles and chicken. But seriously, part of what people value in matchmakers is the vetting we do of our clients. With online dating, nobody is checking out these people for you.

I realize not everyone can afford a matchmaker, and there are a lot of success stories about people who met online, got married, and lived happily ever after. Good for them. There are a lot of crazies online, too. Anyone using match.com, e-harmony, or another online dating site needs to be very careful.

Dating only works when there is honesty and, let's face it, there is an incredible amount of false information on the web. Online dating is no exception. A guy claims he's single, but he's actually married. Or he says he runs a Fortune 500 company, when in fact he cleans its bathrooms. Online man states that he's looking for "the one," but he's really focused on one night—dinner and down. He claims he's tall, but at best he's 5′5″ with shoes on. A survey conducted by Opinion Matters found that over half of Americans who date online lie on their profiles.

Online dating should be a last resort. Give the real world a chance for *at least* six months before clicking your way into the virtual one. Why? In addition to all the blatant lying that happens on dating websites, the Internet allows people to hide behind walls and avoid face-to-face socialization. Meeting a man in person gives you a much better sense of his personality and appearance than an online profile ever will.

I think computers and smart phones are turning people into social idiots. When I was in Bora Bora, one of the most romantic places on Earth, I was disturbed by the behavior of the young honeymooners I saw. Mr. and Mrs. Newlywed were lying on lounge chairs in their poolside cabanas, both staring at the phones in their hands. Is this the image they had in mind of a sexy honeymoon: apps, texts, and web browsing? I mean look at each other, touch each other. You're in paradise with a hot mate. What could possibly be on your phone that is more enticing? Computers and smart phones have their place (on a honeymoon I suggest you power off if you plan to get off!), but they are not an equal substitute for in-person interaction.

I am well aware of how popular online dating is. In early 2014, the U.S. online dating industry had an estimated worth of $2.1 billion, with 40 million Americans participating in it. How can I oppose a practice that is so widespread? Does that make me a dinosaur waiting for an asteroid to take me out of my misery?

Just because something catches on doesn't mean it's superior to everything else. Think of disco. I am not saying that you should never use online dating, just as it's okay to have a guilt-free disco party. But I'm suggesting that you keep online dating strictly as a reserve and if you use it, continue to look around in the real world for Mr. Right. Online dating is one tool in the kit and not the best one. Next chapter I'll talk about precautions to take if you go on a date with a person you met online, but for now let's move on to in-the-flesh pick-up tips.

Pick-Up Tips

I can already sense your resistance. The book is shaking in your nervous hands and you're saying, "Pick-up tips . . . Barbara, are you joking? I can't do that!" Well, let me tell you, missy, when you want something you have to seize it before the opportunity passes. If you're young and expect life to come to you, you'll be waiting for it until your hair turns gray, and then you'll still be waiting! What is the purpose of taking two hours to get ready to go out with your girlfriends if you're just going to sit there with them at a bar and not talk to anyone else? You might as well put on sweats and watch a DVD together at a friend's house. When you're out and about, you can connect with at least one guy. It may not materialize into anything, but it's better than hiding in plain sight. So do yourselves a favor, women of all ages, by feeling your power and taking initiative. Here's how . . .

Lock Eyes and Give Off the Vibe

Eye contact is number-one. When there is someone in a room you're drawn to, try to make eye contact with him. Do a soft glance to get him to look in your direction. Then when he locks eyes with you, smile. Create interest right away with your body language and see if that engages him enough to walk over to you. It's a very simple method but works incredibly well. If he's single and interested, he'll probably make his way toward you.

You want men to feel that they have permission to approach you. You do that by making eye contact and giving off the vibe that you're open to meeting someone. In other words, when you put perfume on, someone will smell it. Too many women give off a cold vibe yet wonder why men don't talk to them. It's not complicated. If you're sending the signal that you're not approachable, most guys will heed the message and stay back. They'll think that flower's been pollinated or sprayed with pesticide, so this bee is moving on to the next one.

Make the Move

I'm a fan of women being assertive and generally believe that women start relationships and end them. When you want something, go for it. Because that moment in time will pass you by. He is going to leave and you're probably never going to see him again. You have to grasp the opportunity. Maybe he's married or in a relationship, but maybe he's not. He may not even know you're there! I think the worst thing you can do is to say nothing and not take any action. Ideally, try to get the guy to come to you, but he might be oblivious, timid, or partially blind, so you may have to move a little closer. If the elliptical machine next to him opens up, get on it and say hi. You want something? Go get it.

You might be thinking that men like to chase things, so if you take away the chase then they're going to lose interest. First of all, that's not always the case. There are men who want a lot of reassurance that a woman is into them. One good-looking, twentysomething guy recently put it this way, "I don't like the chase. I like knowing." He prefers that women approach him because then he knows they're interested and not married. Secondly, just because you make eye contact with a guy and strike up a light-and-lively conversation with him doesn't mean that you've taken the chase away. You've let him know that you'd like to play the game, and you're checking to see whether he wants to join.

In Lake St. Louis, Missouri, women in my mom's housing association thought Mel was really handsome. He was a widower, and many women dropped off casseroles with notes saying, "Enjoy this dish—Molly." My mom, though of the same age, was different from the seventy-some-thing-year-old casserole girls. She went after Mel more assertively. She wrote him a note that invited him to dinner and asked him to call to confirm. Mel dialed her up and said he'd be there. My mom made him chicken and polenta, and just like that they started to date. Now they're married. My mom is like me; she wants to squeeze all she can out of life. But if she had been like all the other ladies dropping off casseroles and hiding behind bushes, Mel might not have noticed her while eating his gloppy dinners alone.

When you can't find a way to get the guy to you, then you have to get to him. What do you say once you've approached?

Use the Gift of Gab

First of all, don't be obnoxious or in a guy's face, sending the message that you're going to own his balls if you're in his life. You don't want to be gutsy to the point that you come across as ridiculous, so just initiate a casual conversation.

One method is to lead with a friendly comment related to your surroundings. "Is it always this busy here? This place is like who's who in the zoo." You just threw him an easy pitch to hit. If he's not wearing a ring, appears interested in you, and keeps the conversation going, then it's time to figure out whether he's single. Some women are comfortable asking this outright. Others want to use a more indirect approach, like "We're going to have a drink at the bar while we're waiting. If you feel up for it, come join us."

Or, let's say you're grocery shopping and you see a fetching fella. You might say, "Hi, I just noticed you grocery shopping, and you don't have a ring on, so I was wondering whether you're single." If that's too gutsy for you, take a less bold approach, like "These cabbages are huge!" See how he responds and keep the exchange going if there's momentum. "Don't you love shopping here? They always have the freshest produce." Feel your power and your confidence.

When you sense an opening and ask whether he's single, he is not going to put you down if he's not attracted to you. He's going to let you off easy with, "Oh, thanks, but I have a girlfriend." He's not going to say, "You're ugly," or "What are you doing in the lettuce department with me?" or "How dare you come up to me and be nice?" No, that's never going to happen. Ever. What you anticipate negatively happening is never going to occur. Get your power. Know who you are and what your attraction levels are. The short, heavy, bald guy who wants the tall, skinny blonde is not being realistic, for instance.

Men love to talk about themselves. They like to open up about who they are, and they thrive on compliments. Test run a compliment on a guy who's a friend or relative and watch as he puffs up like a rooster. It's really kind of incredible to witness. One strategy, then, is to draw a man toward you with a compliment. "I'm sorry, but I just have to let you know that you have the most gorgeous hair of any guy I've seen in a long time." He'll be charmed and start talking to you. Or, "Oh my God, I love how tall you are. In the dating world, it's really hard to find a man as tall as you." While complimenting him, you're throwing it out there that you're dating.

For those of you really shy girls, how about a note? Go back to the 1950s. If you can't say it aloud, you could instead write a message on the back of your card. "Wanting to know if you're single. I am. Any interest? Call me." Walk up to him. Say, "I'd like to give you this. Thank you." Hand him your card (you don't need to work to have a card; just carry one around as a way for people to reach you and remember you by). You'll walk toward your car with a smile on your face. Maybe he'll give you call. Maybe he's not single. Maybe he's not interested. Oh well. Next.

Another tactic is to send a friend over, a wingwoman. She's like the imitation matchmaker who gets the process started or reports back that he's a creep with a squeaky voice.

Get in Their Heads

You could be with a group of women and not be the best-looking one among them, but a man is going to single you out because he likes your positive attitude, your energy, your smile, your take-charge approach. My clients love that kind of woman. What you have you got to lose? I'll tell you what you have to lose: that guy walking out the door who you never connected with.

First Dates

HOPEFULLY YOU'VE UTILIZED YOUR network and have been out on the town smiling and chatting up the chaps, and you've got a date or two lined up. Now you need to learn how to take a levelheaded approach to a first date so that it doesn't feel like a dog-and-pony show. They'll be no stuffing of bras, rants about sleaze-bag ex-boyfriends, or hiccups brought on by four dirty martinis. Let's jump in with a few do's, don'ts, and how-to's.

Drop the Mask and Cut Him Some Slack

When meeting clients for the first time, I ask them to show up in work-out clothes. I don't want to see them when they're all put together, dressed like it's a job interview or five-star restaurant. I favor anything that allows people to get real right away. Unfortunately, the first-date atmosphere is usually the opposite—fake and ridiculous—with count-less decisions about what to wear, numerous calls to friends for advice, and hours spent getting ready. People try so hard to make a good impression on a first date that they don't act like themselves.

I'm a case in point! For my first date with Robert, I got my hair blown out and ironed (certainly not something I do on a daily basis), and I arrived thirty minutes early to his country club, where we were meeting for dinner. Anyone who knows me knows I'm always fifteen minutes late. Robert—ever punctual—was thrilled to see that I got there even earlier than he did. He suggested that we have a bottle of red wine. I hate red wine, but I said yes and drank half of the bottle with him, which is more than I usually consume. As you can tell, I repeatedly misrepresented myself on that first date.

For our next several dates, Robert always arrived bearing a bottle of red wine. I finally had to sit him down and tell him that I actually can't stand the stuff. You can't keep playing games, so it's better not to start. Luckily, Robert was okay about the wine and enough went well during the first month of dating that we made it to where we are today, but it was silly to start the relationship by being fake and trying to please. That was a waste of time. He learned the hard way that my showing up early was a total charade because I probably haven't done it again since!

Misrepresenting ourselves is a very common first-date mistake. Another one is bailing before giving someone a fair shot. People look for outs rather than ins. It's as though they're just waiting for an excuse for why they should not go out on another date. I hear from clients, "Barbara, she was bankrupt ten years ago; I can't deal with that." Or, "he has a receding hairline" or "his teeth need work." I say give it a break if it's something that can be fixed. That's what hairstylists and dentists are for. If a mistake from his past bothers you, does it look like he's learned from it and changed?

People walk away for such ridiculous reasons. I set up a guy, John, with a woman named Kayla. They met at Starbucks and had such a fun time together that they immediately planned another date for later in the week. Before they parted, Kayla told John, "You've got to come meet my dog. He's in the car. I take him everywhere with me." When John approached the car, the dog growled at him and became agitated.

Later that day, Kayla told me what happened and firmly decided, "I cannot go out with anyone my dog doesn't like, which means you're going to have to cancel this date for me." Thinking this was completely cuckoo, I tried talking sense into her, but she kept insisting no, no, no. I called John to cancel the date and told him why. He then called Kayla up and out and said, "I don't believe this for a minute. I have never had a dog not like me." Reluctantly she ended up meeting him that Sunday in a park. It went great, the dog liked him, and Kayla and John are now married to each other! But they almost never went out again because of the dog!

On your first date, keep in mind that you, too, are probably going to be hypercritical—though hopefully you won't use your dog's reaction as a test of character—so allow for a margin of error. The guy might be nervous or trying too hard. Cut him some slack. When there's even the slightest bit of fire on a date, I think that you should go out again. If you're saying to yourself, "I don't know," then give it another chance. The jury is hung for a reason. It's like when you see a movie for the second time and think, wow, I have such a deeper appreciation for this film; I didn't pick up on how great the dialogue was the first time I watched it. Second and third dates can be like that as the guy slowly reveals himself to you, and you begin to notice and appreciate his qualities.

This is why I have a three-date rule for my clients. I almost always try to get them to go out three times with the same person before they make any decisions. Since the first date unfortunately tends to be a bit fake and both people are nervous, it's not a good gauge of compatibility. Secondly, people frequently underestimate the relationship's potential. A common complaint is, "I didn't feel any chemistry with him." If you're under thirty-five, I can buy the chemistry argument, but as you get older, I believe you can develop chemistry. At first, I didn't think Robert and I had chemistry. I stereotyped myself as the girl who worked out who wanted a super fit guy. But the chemistry grew as I witnessed him caring for his quadriplegic brother and his three sons. We'll talk about chemistry more in chapter six, but now that we've established that you need to be yourself and give him a chance, let's move on to the where, when, and how of the first date.

Set It Up

Let's think back to last chapter's crash course on pick-up tips. You're out and about. You meet someone. The conversation is going well, but it's time for you to leave. Tell the guy that you've really enjoyed meeting him. He might take the initiative, suggest a date, and get your number.

Fantastic. Some guys are go-getters and grab the reins. Others are not as bold and want you to give them a more direct sign that you're interested. With those types, you could make a suggestion like, "We should meet for drinks at Take Charge Café. They have super deals on Saturday afternoons and a big outdoor patio." If he perks up and agrees or suggests an alternative, awesome. The guy who just says, "I'll call you," and doesn't set anything up is iffy at best.

If you sense that he's interested in you, try to set up a first date during the pick-up. That's number one. Number two, if you don't know the person and he didn't come recommended to you by someone you trust, make it a daytime date. When people are around and it's light out, there's less to be afraid of. Daytime dates keep things from getting too physical too quickly. No matter how horny the guy is, I doubt he's expecting to score if you're meeting him at 10 a.m. for a latte. Keep the heat in the beverages, and if it's going well, take a stroll downtown (not that downtown!).

I like to think of the first three dates as three stages of presenting yourself. The first date is an informal and careful lead-in. I always suggest stupid, simple first dates, like the example above of meeting at a cafe. This makes you feel safer and less invested in the date. Since you might have met this guy online or after you'd had ten shots of tequila, you first need to establish that you feel comfortable with him and could see yourself giving him a chance. You don't want to give out too much personal information. If he's normal and nice, be friendly but not overly revealing. An easy-breezy first date also allows you to dress in a relaxed fashion. You don't want to start with your best outfit because you can only go downhill from there. Start with a more casual look.

The second date is the build up. If the first date went well enough to warrant the second one, consider scheduling it around an activity, like riding bikes, bowling, hiking, or going to a museum. The key is to get the guy in different environments. Don't have all three dates in restaurants, for example. That's boring, predictable, and only shows you what he's like when he's eating, talking, and sitting down. The third date can be dressy (a fancy dinner, for example) and is the crescendo. If you really like this guy, get your game face on. Wear a nice outfit, be fun, friendly, easy to talk to, and engaging. This is you at your most attentive, attractive, and alluring.

Now that we have an overview of the first three dates, let me slow down and get more detailed. For the first date and until you're comfortable, take your own car. If the guy comes to you fully vetted by a trustworthy source, then you can let him pick you up if you'd like. But if you met the guy online or at a bar, don't let him anywhere near your house. You also don't want to be trapped in his car if it turns out he's narcoleptic or homicidal.

There is nothing wrong with saying to a guy who offers to pick you up, "I'd feel more comfortable meeting you out. I'm sorry to seem skittish, but for my own peace of mind, this is what I have to do until I feel like I've gotten to know you better." Furthermore, if you want to end the date when you find out that at age forty-five he has never lived anywhere except his mother's house, you'll be able to because you have your own wheels. Your car is your exit strategy.

By car, foot, scooter, or piggyback, when you arrive safely at the location of choice the first question is: Is he there? If not, how long did you wait for him to show up? Now I know I've admitted that I tend to run fifteen minutes behind schedule and that's not good. But some of you ladies have kept guys waiting for thirty or forty-five minutes—you know who you are! Well, truthfully, usually when guys experience that, they walk. They can't take it. They see a whole life of that: She doesn't respect my time. She's self-consumed. If she's like this about time, she's going to be like this in other aspects. I'm never going to feel important.

By being very late, the woman is sending those signals. And she'll say to me, "For God's sake, Barbara, I had a valid excuse for being late." She'll sell herself on the idea that she doesn't really want that kind of guy anyway. "If he gets all bent out of shape about a few minutes here and there—I mean I called him, I texted him, I told him I was going to be late. That's his problem." Okay, fine. Maybe you miss out on a wonderful guy because of your hardheadedness. It's give and take. You like that he's corporate America and successful. Part of his success is probably due to the fact that he's punctual with his clients every day and responsible. Therefore, my suggestion is to be on time (or very close to it!).

When he sees you, how excited does he look? If you lock eyes and he gives you a big, open-mouthed yawn, that's not a good sign. Does he get up to say hi or stay seated at the table? How is he dressed? Is he neat? Do you like his style? Does it match up well with yours? He's in boardshorts and flipflops. You're in heels and a dress. Maybe that's fine with you; maybe it's not. Always be observant. Take in the data and analyze it.

Read His Lips

After the first once-over (his excitement level, his appearance, and so forth), the conversation will be the next major test. Say hi and be pleasant. Once you guys are nicely arranged (he's bought your latte, for instance, and you're seated at the table), he should ask you lots of questions and not just talk about himself the whole time. I hate it when guys go on and on about themselves. It doesn't matter what the storyline is, you don't matter and never will because he hasn't asked now and he won't later. Does he talk over you? You want a guy who is attentive, polite, and respectful of your opinions. At the same time, be sure that you're not dominating the conversation. Take a breath when you're talking. Slow down if you think you're getting excited and blabbering away.

Ask him pertinent questions without making the date like a job interview. You can do that by leading into the subject gently. "Did you come here straight from work?" Let's say he did and he mentions an aspect of his job. Inquire about that and how he likes working there. As the conversation goes on, get a handle on how he feels about his success in life or lack thereof. Was there lots of grumbling about a jerky boss, or does he love his job and show pride in his achievements?

Get an idea of how he's living and whether it's compatible with the lifestyle you want. Let's say he lives in a messy, cramped apartment with two other guys. If he's twenty-two, that might be fine with you, but if he's fifty-seven, realize that you might have to become a sugar mama if you continue to date. Ask him what he did over the weekend. That will reveal a lot. Bachelor weekend in Vegas with lots of details unrevealed or dinner with his two-year-old daughter and a Sunday spent fishing on the lake? Depending on where you are in your life and what you value, you're going to find these kinds of details to be green lights or red flags.

How long has it been since he was in a relationship? If he hasn't been in one for five years, he probably doesn't want one. If he tells you he looks forward to coming home to an empty house (I know a guy who said this), take the big fat hint and realize he doesn't want a serious relationship.

Did any subject come up that could be problematic down the line? Let's say he noted that he hunts, and you're not sure how you feel about that. Store all this information away.

Don't get too personal. Be informative about what you like to do and how you spend a typical weekend, for instance. Keep the conversation casual, like, "You know that new sushi restaurant on 4th Street? My friend went there and raved about it. I'd like to try it some time. Do you like sushi?"

People talk about taking baby steps. On a first date, I believe you should give out baby pieces of information. All good things in all good time. Don't tell the guy that you had hemorrhoid surgery last week. Some of you will say, "But, Barbara, I want to be honest." You're not being dishonest; you're being context appropriate. Be yourself and be animated, but choose laidback topics. After all, you wouldn't tell strangers your personal information, and in most cases the man you're having your first date with is a stranger. Don't tell the guy how you had $30,000 in credit card debt or that you knew it was time to file for divorce when you had reoccurring dreams about running over your ex-husband with his precious car.

As I mentioned before, it's really not a good idea to talk extensively about previous relationships on first dates. The guy might ask about your last relationship, which is fine, but keep your response brief. Don't start telling him you had your heart broken after your ex cheated on you with the manager of the local dry cleaner. You always wondered why he liked to have his shirts starched so often and then one day . . . No, don't go there. In general, restrain yourself from getting into a runaway monologue of too much personal information. Hold onto yourself a little bit. Women should be slightly mysterious to a man, not a sponge that, when squeezed, releases all its contents.

Also, whatever you do, do NOT tell men your future relationship plan as in: "So after the dry-cleaning fiasco, I realized I'm thirty-five and single. I need to get the ball in motion and get married before the end of the year." He doesn't even know you, but you're already plotting out his life. That's a big turnoff to guys. They'll think that you don't want them because of who they are but for what they can provide. Along the same lines, don't rant and rave about what you can't stand about men, relationships, or life. You will drive him crazy and not in the good way.

During the conversation, use your sense of humor. Men love that. The most beautiful woman on season 17 of the TV show *The Bachelor* got cut. She was also the most verbal about loving him. What did she lack? The remaining contestants were more spontaneous and had a sense of humor. She was very serious and had a hard time letting go of control. If you're not funny, at least celebrate his sense of humor and show that you like to laugh and can take a joke.

Energy is extremely important. You can't be a bore on a date. You might not be that interesting right now and should find ways to make yourself more engaging. Increase the excitement level in your life, as we talked about in chapter two, in order to be your most captivating self.

During the date, be mentally there. Don't be thinking about what your kids are doing that night or what your client's reaction was to the email you sent. Distraction is not an inviting quality. It sends the signal that you don't value the guy's time and that he can't keep your attention.

Let Him Treat

On the first date and beyond, the guy should treat. He should grab the bill with no hesitation. If you split the bill on the first date, you'll be reaching for your wallet for the rest of your life. You'll be the halfsie girl. Some of you are going to find this old-fashioned, and that's okay, but my opinion is let the guy be a guy. Let him be chivalrous. After a few dates, you can buy the movie tickets or handle the cab fare, but let him pay for dinner.

I don't think women should pick up tabs at restaurants. Once you start splitting the bill, it becomes a pattern. Men like routines and want to know what their routines are going to be, so don't establish one that later you'll want to break. All that being said, don't bleed the poor guy dry. Be sensitive to what he can afford. It helps, especially in the beginning, to let him make the final decision of where to go for the date. He doesn't have to take you to an expensive restaurant. What about a picnic? The amount he spends on you is not what matters. What matters is that he is generous with what he has. When I ask women what trait they just cannot tolerate in a guy, many will say cheapness.

In my opinion, chivalry should not be dead. To really feel like a woman—to be courted and cherished—is timeless. The personal intimacy of a hand-written card or flowers tells you that you are appreciated. The old-fashioned values need to come back: men opening doors for women, holding their coats. I like it when a guy orders at least part of the meal for me, such as the drinks. It shows that he can take charge. But it all depends on what *you* want. If you like to take charge and order the meal, that's great. Whatever it is that you want, don't sell out on it. Stay true to yourself.

More Do's and Don'ts on the First Date

Trust your instincts. Whenever you sense that something is off about a guy—you get the feeling that he's not who he claimed he was or he just gives you a creepy feeling—don't wait around to confirm that suspicion. Come up with an excuse why you need to leave, and get out of there. Often women wonder if they're being too hard on someone. That can be the case if they like everything about him except for wishing he was wearing a cuter shirt. But if the guy sets off your shadar—your radar for spotting shady characters—you're not being mean; your instincts are kicking in to say "danger, danger."

I know a wealthy man named Tim who recently met a woman from Montana online. They Skype and talk on the phone and have never met in person. She wants to come to San Diego and stay with him for two weeks and is already talking about moving here. She's in between jobs and renting a place with tons of roommates. I'm like, yoo-hoo, Tim? Anyone home? At best this woman is looking for a rescue mission. At worst, she's certifiable or a scam artist. If a person's behavior strikes you as strange, trust your instincts and protect yourself.

For that matter, *stay local*. I don't think it's advisable to go beyond the area where you live to meet people. San Diegans who expand their search to L.A., Las Vegas, and Phoenix, for example, can't control their dating situation. Whenever you venture off your home turf, you are vulnerable. However, if you live in a remote area, you might find that you have to drive a little ways to date new people, but choose meeting places you're familiar and comfortable with.

Filter and chill. If you haven't been in a relationship for a long time and you've been mostly hanging out with women, you've gotten used to not filtering what you say. Women are often forgiving of each other. Oh, I really didn't mean that. Okay, fine. Men, on the other hand, hang on every word. Some women are so brash and blunt on their initial dates that the guy will call me and say, "She's just too hardcore for me. It was funny at first, but after a couple of dates with her, I couldn't take it. She's really got an edge." The edge is not real. It's a safety zone; she's trying to protect herself and not waste any time because she's been hurt before. But it's hard to convince guys of that, which means you need to be careful about the type of guard you put up. The way to protect yourself is to hold onto yourself: don't divulge compromising personal information or get physical right away.

Don't give up the goods. I know women who got too hot and heavy too soon because they "immediately clicked" with their date. I cannot stand that expression. You didn't immediately click anything, except three glasses of wine. The guy's holding your hand, putting his arm around you, and you're starting to daydream. It's called attraction. Sometimes we begin to think from the neck down and the brain takes a vacation; it's strolling down the beach looking for a margarita. The guy's drawing you in and you think you really want to kiss him. Do a choke-chain on yourself. Wake up real quick. If this is a man you don't know, especially if it's some random guy you met online, don't start making out, because you'll have nothing left. If you lead with your physical attributes, what remains? That should be the dessert, but he's on a diet and can't have it yet.

You want to lead with your mind and your presence. Find out if you've got common ground before you give any ground. A man's agenda is often short term. It's fine with me if yours is too, but you're probably not looking for advice from me on how to pull off a one-night stand. That's pretty easy to accomplish, and you'll find a lot of guys who will gladly fulfill that task. But if you're looking for a serious relationship, slow things down on the physical front. I don't suggest anything more than one light kiss (if that!) on a first date. And never ever go back to a guy's house if you're hoping that it could become a relationship. You're sending the signal that sex is on the evening's program, and it will be hard to reprogram his expectations once you're there.

Don't overdo the makeup. I'll tell a client that the woman he's going to meet is naturally beautiful. Then she shows up with her face coated in so much makeup that a geisha would do a double take. Ladies, if you look in the mirror and are startled, imagine what his reaction is going to be. Be as close to who you are as possible. If you don't wear eye shadow ninety percent of the time, don't put it on for a date. You'll feel like it's Halloween, and freaky is not the look you're going for. Besides, if you continue dating him you'll eventually return to the way you normally wear your makeup, so why show him a false image?

Boob overkill is a big no-no. Don't push your breasts up so high that they touch your nose when you look down at the menu. If you pad and push yourself up to a size DD, your chest is going to look like an apparatus that's been strapped on to your body. Secondly, if you end up seeing this guy beyond the first few dates, think how bummed he's going to be when he pulls that bra and padding off and discovers they've been covering little eggs. The main thing to think about is: What are you trying to promote about yourself? If you're promoting brains, you'll see if he has any. If you're highlighting that chest of yours, you're basically telling him that sex kitten has arrived.

Do a simple background check. Before your date, ask the guy where he works and try to verify it through an online search. He might be telling you he's a big-shot investment banker, but if he's slow to tell you the name of the company when you ask, he could be lying. Even if you only know one verifiable fact about the person, it validates that he's at least partially truthful.

If you don't know the guy, *don't let him walk you to your car* because you have no idea what he intends to do. Park your car in a well-lit place. You're a big girl. You don't need him to escort you back to it. I know a woman who went on a date with a guy she met online. He said he was from Los Angeles and a professional basketball player. It was all lies. After the date, the man walked her to her car, grabbed the keys from her, and pressed himself against her. When she told him to back off, he seized her throat. She struggled with him and, luckily, was able to get away. You can encounter really scary situations with men you don't know. Let's all just drink chamomile tea and watch DVDs. No, I'm not trying to frighten you; I want you to realize you need to be careful and can't assume that everyone is telling the truth or has good intentions.

If you've had a fun date and the guy offers to walk you to your car, let him know that you enjoyed your time with him and look forward to seeing him again but that you're more comfortable walking by yourself. If that offends him, then the guy's a control freak and you don't want to date him again anyway.

Watch the booze. Alcohol is a social lubricant that can get you over the jitters, but too much of it will have you slurring your words and guffawing at his jokes. Know your tolerance and don't push it. Watch his booze intake as well. If he's slamming back the drinks and not the age of a frat boy, that could be a bad sign.

Make a follow-up date easy to schedule. Assuming that the date has gone well and you'd like more time to get to know the guy, make it simple to plan a second date. There is a lot of misinformation out there about how women shouldn't make themselves too available to men. Granted, if a guy hasn't called you to follow up for a second date, and a couple of weeks have passed without a word when suddenly he texts you, "Hey, I'm in your neighborhood with some friends. Want to come join me?" I would tell him that you've relocated to Iowa. You don't want to be at someone's beck and call by immediately establishing a pattern that it's okay for him to blow you off since you'll be available whenever he wants you. No, that's lame and you shouldn't put up with his self-centered behavior.

But if a guy sincerely asks you to go out again, don't come up with bogus reasons why your schedule is sooo busy. That's silly and you wouldn't want him to do that to you. Are you hoping he's going to stay in a little box that you can store on a shelf and dust off when you feel like it? Good luck with that plan.

Lastly, in the words of Oscar Wilde, "Be yourself; everyone else is already taken." *Be yourself.* I cannot emphasize that point enough! Your uniqueness is your most powerful asset and will draw matches to you. As we will discuss in the next chapter, you want to make sure the attraction goes beyond good looks and that the two of you are compatible on many levels.

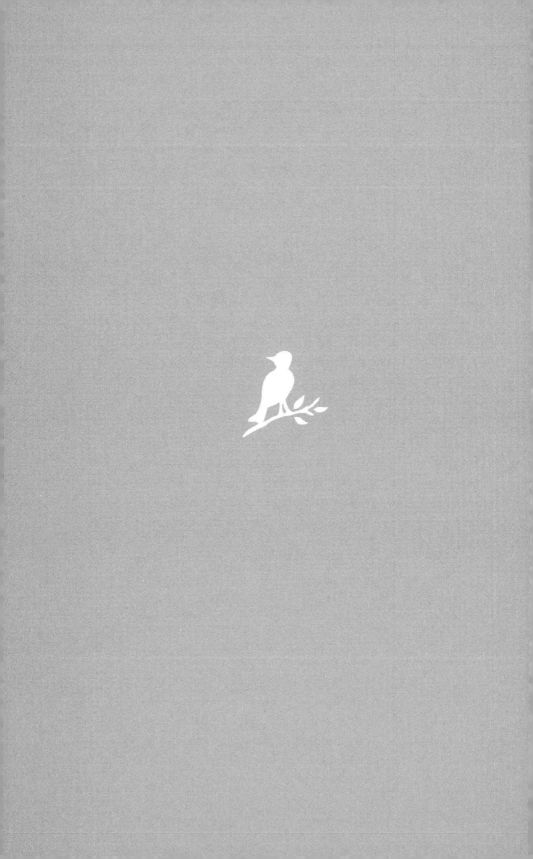

Attraction vs. Compatibility: How Important Are Looks?

WHEN I HAD AN OFFICE, I hated spending Monday mornings in it. Why? Clients would call complaining about their first dates over the weekend. I'd be on the line with one client, while my assistant got a call from a different one. I'd have her mouth to me the name of the person and give me a thumbs up or down so that I could be prepared to take the call. One of the chief complaints was the lack of attraction or chemistry.

Now, keep in mind my three-date rule. I like clients to go on three dates because I believe attraction can grow and chemistry can be created. It's all about giving the person time to reveal his personality, values, and perspectives to you.

First of all, what is attraction? It's something that kindles our interest and draws us to someone. It doesn't have to be about looks. It could be a person's way of being, how he carries himself, takes charge, is affectionate, etc. You could be more attracted to a short, bald guy with a lot of spunk than a fit, thick-haired guy who's boring.

What creates attraction? Chemistry. And what is chemistry? I think of it as how you feel when you're with someone. The *New Oxford American Dictionary* defines chemistry as "the complex emotional and psychological interaction between two people." In my opinion, chemistry can be cultivated. I know some people will fight me on that point, especially the ones who are fixated on looks. Well, imagine this. Let's say you have a couple of dates with a teacher whose appearance doesn't blow you away, but then on the third date he shows you a video of him working with his fifth-grade students, who clearly adore him. I'm sure that new perspective will change the chemistry you feel toward him. You might start picturing yourself raising children with him, which will quickly increase the attraction level. Compare that scenario to Mr. Drop-Dead-Gorgeous who tells you that children are annoying and he just wants to have fun. Do you think you will still be attracted to him in three years when you're pushing for children and he is dragging his feet?

TDHA Syndrome

Women need to overcome the TDHA syndrome—the tendency to be drawn to tall, dark, and handsome assholes. I often find that the really good-looking guys haven't had to develop their other qualities, which can lead them to be unkind or one-dimensional. Their attitude is: all I have to do is shower and show up. The guys who aren't as blessed in the looks department work to make themselves desirable in other ways—with their intelligence, a sense of humor, a depth of caring and responsibility, creativity, and so forth.

The extremely good-looking guys often think someone better is coming around the corner, so if you start dating one, you might find yourself looking over your shoulder in fear. Many women will believe they're not good enough for Mr. Handsome. The relationship starts and ends that way. If you think he's a prize based solely on physical appearance and you don't feel as though you deserve that prize, you might be self-conscious throughout your entire relationship.

Marriage founded primarily on attraction and sex usually goes sideways. The people with the good looks and the strong sexual attraction have the kids right away, the passion fizzles out, and then they're like, now what? Over time, you're not going to want to hop into bed when there's no respect. On the flip side, respect and understanding create chemistry.

Ask yourself if your attraction to a new guy is driven almost completely by his physical appearance. Don't forget about that Dream Match

List I first suggested you draw up in chapter three. A big dating mistake is tossing out all the other important stuff you're looking for just because the guy is hot. Over time, looks fade while character endures.

Good looks can actually lead to problems. There are a lot of attractive men out there who need to be constantly adored. As soon as women drop off that adjective wagon—you're so sexy, strong, etc.—he's on the lookout for the next woman who will dote on him (either during your relationship or after it). When you start dating a man, make sure he's more than gorgeous and not in need of around-the-clock praise. Whatever you do, don't feed that need even more. You'll truly create a monster. If he's hot, he knows it. It's not that you can't compliment him, but don't overdo the praise of his appearance. If you stoke his vanity, you will regret it later, because he will expect you to keep doing it ad nauseam. Men should be rewarded for their good behavior. "Thanks for barbecuing; this chicken is delicious!" or "I really appreciate you cleaning my car."

Over time, life kicks in and you'll get tired of telling Mr. Hot High-Maintenance how wonderful he is, and he might start searching for a duplicate of the sappy girlfriend you once were. When men chase after younger women, sometimes it has to do with the fact that they're trying to regain the way the relationship was. The younger woman reminds the guy of how it felt before the boredom and nagging began, for example.

It is very important to be aware of the precedents you set in the beginning of a relationship. Men are creatures of habit and establish routines quickly. Don't be too pleasing with Mr. Sexy because he'll get used to it, take advantage of you, and then probably get rid of you.

But it's not just about him. It's about your self-perception. Some women are attracted to cheaters, for example. They pride themselves on the fact that "he always comes back to me." Well, whoopty-do. I can't tell you how often I hear, "I'm still the women he loves. The affairs didn't mean anything to him." They didn't? He just got naked and stuck his body parts into a different person, but it didn't mean anything at all? Or I'll hear, "He couldn't help himself." Please. Do you think he would see it that way if you were cheating on him?

Take a cold shower. Wake yourself up. Why don't you think you deserve better? If you've stayed with guys who have cheated on you repeatedly or made you feel insecure about what you bring to the table, you need to take a good hard look at yourself and figure out why you keep doing this. Is being seen with the sexy guy worth it if he's running around on you? Wouldn't it be better to be with a loving, respectful man?

I think of my mother and how when she saw my father for the first time, she told her friend she was going to marry him. My father was model handsome—a prize that my mother wanted to win. But the plan backfired because my mom had low self-esteem and didn't see herself on his level as far as looks were concerned. She became subservient and waited on him, the king of the castle, hand and foot. It was as if she thought he was doing her a favor. My mom lost her power in the relationship, and my father cheated on her, which was really a blessing in disguise because that gave her the motivation to go out and make it on her own. She became a company executive and a strong woman. When my dad came crawling back to make amends, she told him, "Don't let the door hit you on the ass on the way out." My mom would have stayed squashed if the affair never happened and the marriage had continued. You have to be careful about what you wish for sometimes—what you think is a win quickly becomes a loss.

Beauty is the true core of a person. It emanates from within. I'm not saying that looks aren't important, because they are (more on this in a moment), but too often women overlook great guys because they aren't as traditionally attractive as Big Ego. Or, they're drawn to total losers who are underemployed and irresponsible but incredibly good-looking. The ideal situation is to find a guy who is physically attractive *and* has other desirable traits that are on your list.

You could make a balding guy with a winning personality feel so good about himself that he decides to throw out the toupee and rock the baldness. We are capable of giving those we love a lot of confidence. It works the other way, too; look for the guy who allows you to drop your own armor and be yourself. That's going to feel better over time than the guy who always gives you the impression that you're just barely meeting his requirements. Insecurity is a relationship killer.

Fixers and Projects

It's common to be attracted to people with whom we are not compatible. That is a big problem in relationships. It's not just looks and sex appeal that derail us from what we want, but also "projects."

Lots of women are attracted to the underdog guy. They want to make his life better. Women enjoy making a difference; they like to play nurse and problem solve. If they've never had children, this guy becomes their "child." They feed off of him being the problem guy, because it gives them a sense of control and allows them to tap their nurturing side, which they love to use. People say it's lonely at the top. It's hard to make your way into the power guy's control tower. It's easier to take the guy who needs you. Women make sure the underdog has money in his bank account, is laying off the booze, or whatever the issue is. He's a project. She's the fixer. And that's the main attraction.

Those kinds of guys are sweet puppy dogs and usually good in bed. They need to have a strong card, right? They know how to reward women sexually, but they're usually not going to stay, and they're usually not going to resolve whatever ails them (such as drinking, drugs, unemployment, or anger).

Can these guys get it together? Sometimes. Some of them need a reason to work hard or get rid of bad habits, and the nurturing woman becomes that motivation. Behind every great man is a great woman, as the saying goes. More often than not, though, the "project" ends in frustration, because people don't change unless they want to. You can't force anyone to stop drinking, for instance. The alcoholic has to recognize that he has a problem and have the willpower to stop drinking and move his life in a different direction. Women tend to want to try, try, and try again, so it's important to set time limits. Otherwise, you can waste several years on a dysfunctional "fixer" relationship.

If you're the fixer and he's the new project, give the puppy-dog-on-the-couch/tiger-in-the-sack a chance, but not for long. I say three months. At that point, if you haven't seen tangible improvement, let go and give the project back to him. He'll find another fixer to glom onto, and around and around he'll go unless he pulls his life together.

If you've been down that dead-end road a few too many times, catch yourself while you're dating. Don't go for the guy with the problems. Hold out for a stable and responsible one. Women are creatures of habit, too, and we repeat our mistakes. Find a different outlet for your inner caretaker. Let her volunteer or work with actual children, for example.

I once had a client named Donna, a successful lawyer who kept dating hot underachievers—boy toys. They were a lot younger than Donna and would live in her house and maintain the pool. Because of her control issues, she didn't attract movers and shakers. After awhile, though, she got tired of being with the boy toys and hired me as her matchmaker. I set her up with Tom, a successful sales guy with money and personality. It was rocky; they broke up a number of times because of Donna's difficulty in letting go of control, but eventually they worked things out and got married. Tom could challenge and inspire Donna in a way that the boy toys could not, and that made a meaningful difference in her life.

Whatever hasn't worked for you in past relationships, learn from it and change. It's uncomfortable but vital. Change is risky, but it is a thousand times better than staying stuck. Attract your dream man or get rid of the one you have who went from dream to snooze fest or nightmare. What kinds of guys have you been attracted to who weren't compatible with you? Watch for those signs and break those patterns!

Where do you want to go next? You always have to ask yourself that question, whether it's a next step or a next person. Look to the future, ladies, and don't drag past mistakes with you.

The Importance of Appearances

As much as I believe that compatibility is far more important than physical appearance for cultivating a healthy, happy relationship, I'm not going to lie and say that looks don't matter, because they do. They matter a lot. His looks and yours. As my hairdresser says, "Men are visual animals. Women are emotional ones."

If you haven't realized it by now, I'm big on self-improvement. It's important to take care of ourselves inside and out. We need to eat well, exercise, learn, socialize, and do whatever it takes to have healthy minds and bodies. We all want to be loved, and we're all looking for direction for improvement. The trouble comes when women start listening to what other people say or want without thinking for themselves. If you love your long hair, for example, don't take the advice of the person who suggests that you cut it short. Before we get too far along in this section, I want to make it very clear that *you must be yourself* and look how you want to look. Don't sell yourself out.

At the same time, every woman wants to improve her appearance, whether it's losing ten pounds, reducing the oiliness of her skin, or making her wardrobe more current. Everyone is insecure about something. Identify what it is about your appearance that you want to work on and then work on it. Don't just think about it. Execute. Like anything, to get positive results you have to invest time and energy. While working on that area of improvement, I highly suggest that you accentuate the assets in your appearance, whether it's your eyes, legs, lips, or another attribute.

If you aren't sure how to go about improving or accentuating your physical form, ask for advice. Do you have a female friend who always looks very well put together? She has an eye for style and color and would probably be really flattered if you turned to her for advice. People enjoy sharing their expertise and helping others. You could consult with salespeople at makeup counters or clothing stores. Women's magazines have helpful tips, too. Personal trainers can establish workout routines and nutritional plans for you. Personal training can be expensive, so if you're on a tight budget, just get two or three sessions. If you don't have money, try to barter. Let's say you know a personal trainer who has two young children. Offer to babysit them in exchange for training sessions. There is no excuse for not taking steps toward self-betterment. When you're willing, you can always find a way to get started.

If you don't care about yourself, then why would you expect another person to? You want to be in a good place mentally and physically when you're dating. That way you'll draw men who also value their minds and bodies. For those of you already in a relationship, think about what a dose of self-improvement could do for your self-worth as well as your relationship.

Eat Healthy and Move

Because most women want to get in better physical shape, which usually happens by eating better and exercising more, I'd like to take a moment to offer advice on this subject. First of all, I don't like the word "dieting." To lose weight, start to eat healthy foods in sensible portions. Think colorful plates. Have a piece of protein with vegetables and whole grains. The whole no-carb thing is silly. You need carbohydrates, just like you need any other type of food.

The other part to losing weight and getting fit is exercise. People often say that they don't have enough time to exercise. If that's the case, get in ten minutes here and ten minutes there. Pretty soon you'll have thirty minutes for the day. People aren't moving enough. They're sitting too much because of the way we work, commute, and watch TV for entertainment. We're always on our butts. Mankind wasn't made to be this sedentary, and a sitting-around lifestyle is not good for us. Get moving. Walk, jog, join a gym, take fitness classes, play a sport—whatever interests you—but do something. Exercise is vital to your overall well-being.

Losing weight can be hard, but it's worth it to have more energy and be able to wear that cute skirt that's been sitting in the closet for two years. Food can be used to celebrate, of course, but if you've noticed that you're packing on the pounds, maybe food has become too much of a reward or overindulgence. Try to think of eating as energy creation that backfires when overdone. However, once a week allow yourself to eat whatever you want. It will ease the transition. After adopting healthy habits, you might not even want to reach for those cookies anymore or may learn to enjoy smaller portions of sweets.

With the help of a medical professional, decide how many calories a day you should be consuming. Then, start making your choices based on numbers. You can have that donut or two glasses of wine, but you can't have them all, especially if you're over thirty-five. I will never recommend that anyone starve herself to lose weight. That's a really bad idea, and it doesn't work. Order the French toast you love, just don't eat four slices of it in one sitting.

Trying to be your best weight and your best self takes a lot of discipline. My advice is don't attempt to change everything all at once. Let's say you love dessert. If you're eating it four times a week, start by cutting back to two times a week. If you generally have never liked exercise, begin by scheduling a morning walk three days a week. When changes are too drastic, we revolt by quitting, and then we feel frustrated with ourselves. Be patient. Weight loss happens gradually. When you see ads or articles touting the latest way to lose fifteen pounds in one month, roll your eyes and move on. Anything that sounds too easy and too good to be true is not true, so don't waste your time on false promises.

Here are a few more healthy eating tips:

- Don't eat stuff in cans. It's too salty. Lots of women put on water weight because their food is high in sodium.

- Get in the habit of putting food on your plate. When it's gone, it's gone, and don't reach for more. Some families eat country style in which tons of food is put into bowls and placed in the center of the table for everyone to grab. That's not a good way to control how much you consume.

- At a restaurant, eat half of the food you're served and take the other half home.

- Soda—give it up or buy the truly natural kind.

- Drink more water. If you don't like drinking water, add fresh peaches, a lemon wedge, or any other natural ingredient that makes it more exciting for you.

♦ If your schedule is really busy, on Sunday cook a bunch of food all at once and use it throughout the week, like sweet potatoes, broccoli—be sure not to overcook it, though—and salmon. Cook a big batch of protein, such as chicken or fish, that you can use throughout the week (e.g., chicken salad, chicken with vegetables, chicken soup).

Make sure that whatever you do, you do it for you, not a guy. I went to a girls' night dinner recently with three other women. Two of them commented on how their husbands wanted them to be thinner, so when the waiter came to take our order, they ordered one ravioli appetizer and one Caesar salad for the entire table. I ventured, "Does someone want to pick out an entrée?" They said, "Oh, no, we're fine. This is plenty." They're practically starving themselves in order to fit the image their husbands want for them. That is not the way to approach weight loss. Do it for yourself and in a sensible way.

Doormat Girls and Balloon Boobs

In the times we live, we can pretty much get whatever we want if we have the money: thicker hair, larger breasts, smoother faces. Look at what just wearing Spanx does for women. But no one has to go buy the best beauty products on the market or get plastic surgery or work out for three hours a day. It's all about choices. Just make sure that whatever you do or don't do, it's *your* choice and no one else's.

Don't be a doormat girl. I try to counsel women to right away, when they see a red flag in a relationship, address it and make a kind request. Give a man a chance, but make some comments. Express yourself about what will work, what won't, and what you might be open to. There are women who will pretty much say and do whatever they think the guy wants.

I've seen young women who had good self-esteem about their body types meet guys who are really into chests, and next thing you know the guys are paying for the women to get breast implants. Now she's got these humongous boobs and she's saying to herself, "I don't really like these breasts." What happened that made her lose sight of who she is? It's almost like women enter a cult in their twenties to forties. Hopefully after fifty you can shake the marbles and they all set within the little holes, like the game. But when you're young those marbles can just bounce around.

Well, what happens is something like this: The guy shows up with the nice clothes and the expensive sports car and says, "Honey, let's go to Vegas for the weekend." The woman's blown away by the money and lifestyle and pretty soon she's hearing, "Don't you love the way that girl in the magazine looks? God, I love chests like that." Oh, you do, she thinks. Oh, really? After more comments like that from him, she's waking up from anesthesia with big balloons on her chest. She hates raw fish, but all of a sudden she's eating in every sushi restaurant in the county because he loves sushi.

She used to always wear jeans and cute sweaters and now he's taken her to Victoria Secret and she's got the double-padded bra and sexy lingerie and is running around the house with her navel hanging out. She's wearing more eye makeup and longer fingernails and has become sex kitten in the last three months. You want to take a scraper and go, yoo-hoo, where are you in there?

We're talking about the power guy here, and once his project is done—the boobs, the makeup, the hair, and the cute clothes—the girl has no power or identity of her own. She's not exciting. She hasn't used her brain in a hell of a long time, and pretty soon she's toast. He no longer wants to shine that trophy, and he's going to go out and find another one until he meets the girl who says, "You know what, I think it's great that you like big chests, but I'm not doing anything to my chest. I like my breasts. And I don't like sushi; I'll go to the restaurant with you and order food that's cooked." I know that men like strong women. I've seen it over and over again in my career. I don't mean strong as in someone who controls him, but strong in that she takes control over her own decisions and doesn't let anyone push her around.

I ran into a girl about six months ago who used to be very cute and petite. This time she had an enormous chest. I looked at her sideways and said, "Katie, what did you do different?" She goes, "Don't start." She touched her breasts and said she knew it was a bad idea. She went out with a guy who paid for her to have her boobs done in L.A. I asked, "Are you still with him?" The answer was no. They're never still with the guy who bought the boobs. The guys who buy the boobs don't stick around.

Now, if you had it in your mind before you met a man that you always wanted to have your breasts done and he says, "Honey, listen, I would love to give that to you as a gift," then that's a great guy because he's going to let you control your decisions and your body, and he's being generous. It's your idea and you pick the surgeon and decide what to do. There's no guarantee that the guy's going to stay in your life, but it's a gift and it's done on a voluntary basis. That's a big distinction. He's not trying to sculpt you into someone you don't want to be.

Now, I'm not saying you can never listen to a partner's requests. Let's say your boyfriend says, "You look hot in skirts. I think you should wear them more often." He's complimenting you and, hey, you probably do look good in skirts and could wear them more frequently. But don't react like, "Okay, sweetie, whatever you want," and then throw out all your pants. No. It's a give and take. You might want your guy to dress better. You wouldn't command him to do so, but at the same time you wouldn't like it if he refused to do anything about it. Maybe you could say, "You look so good in blue. Let's get you a nice blue shirt for that dinner party on Saturday." It's all in the presentation. Be respectful and you'll get respect in return.

Plastic Surgery

I wouldn't live without it. I am fighting aging every step of the way. I told one plastic surgeon just before the anesthesia took me under, "When you think you have my neck as tight as you can get it, give it another jerk." My neck was numb for like six months. That's all right, because I refuse to wear turtlenecks forever.

Why is plastic surgery becoming more common? In part because men are idiots. They'll go on a date and think, wow, this woman is really aging well. They don't realize she's had work done. When you see a woman over fifty who you think looks fabulous for her age, it's likely that she's taken a trip to a plastic surgeon.

Like anything else recommended in this chapter to improve our attractiveness to others, plastic surgery should be about you. If you want it, go for it. Don't ever be convinced by someone else to have work done that you don't want. My mother is eighty-seven and her husband is not going anywhere except into the dirt, so why does she have work done? Because she likes the way she looks and the way it makes her feel. I come from a long line of vain women. My grandmother never saw a mirror she didn't adore, and she could command attention from men. When my grandfather died, she remarried a man two years younger than my father (her son).

Everyone likes to look better, men included. Men get work done, too. For example, they'll have pectoral muscles implanted in their chests or their eyes done. In my opinion, it's not right or wrong; it's all about individual choices. If a woman thinks her eyelids are droopy and unattractive and their appearance really bothers her, why is there anything wrong with working on those eyelids? I'm not pushing plastic surgery for everyone. But I'm a fan of having choices.

I'll tell you one thing, though. As you get older, you can't do anything about sagging skin, especially in your arms. That skin's going to tell you to piss off. If there were a way to firm up the pancake arms that we women get as we age, there would be lines around the block. In the meantime, if it takes rubber bands to pull up the skin on my arms, I'm going to do it because like I said, I'm fighting aging every step of the way.

A good plastic surgeon doesn't change your looks and doesn't talk you into having a surgery that you're uncomfortable with. Let's say you want your eyes done, but he says the rest of you will look old; therefore you should do the whole face. That's bogus and you should move on to the next doctor.

When you're young, you can let your boobs hang out of your shirt and your butt hang out of your shorts. Then as you get older, you're told not to show too much skin, wear longer shorts and higher-cut tops, and that after fifty you shouldn't have long hair. Lame! No, do what you want and what you think looks good. Women limit themselves with this ridiculous "age-appropriate" advice. I hate that expression. Think of yourself as young and spirited. Don't sell yourself into the grave.

You might say, "I'm not into plastic surgery, hair, makeup, the latest clothes, and so forth. What you see is what you get." Wonderful, I applaud you. Your confidence is commendable, and you will attract a person who has a similar perspective. Again, it's all about choices and finding the right match for you.

Now it's time to turn the lights down low and light some candles, because we're about to talk about you know what . . .

Sooner or Later, the Clothes Are Gonna Come Off

EVERYONE HAS A DIFFERENT IDEA of what a great sex life is. I say it's whatever works for you, as long it's also desirable to your partner. Is it a sex life or a sex death? Does it give you life and passion? If it's not mutual or enjoyable, it's a sex death. When it comes to intimacy, there are all kinds of things a person could get into—or not. I think the most important thing sex-wise is matching up with someone who has similar wants. If you're all about the leather and restraints and that makes him want to run to his momma, it's just not going to work. You'll be bored; he'll be scared. Next!

I'll never forget the phone call I got from a woman who had gone on a date with a criminal defense attorney. He wanted to bring his dog in on the action (yes, you read that right). To make matters even worse, he had a Great Dane. The woman wanted no part of either of them and got out of there faster than a boozebag through a dry town.

Let's take a look at some of the questions and quandaries that the bedroom brings up for single and married people.

The First Question . . .

When should you have sex for the first time in a new relationship?

A friend of mine says, "Wait until you've had three drinks." I guess two drinks are just not quite enough to get the job done. Other people, of course, believe you shouldn't have sex until marriage. There's no right or wrong answer. You have to follow your heart and values in deciding.

Let's start with the fast movers. If you're a free spirit who jumps in bed the first night, then that's the card you have going for yourself. You won't know if the guy's continuing to see you because he thinks you're superb in bed or because he likes you or because you're a free ride until he finds Ms. Right, who doesn't go for it as quickly. Some couples had sex on the first night and have been together ever since, but most of the time I don't find that to be the case. In general, when you're looking for a serious relationship, it's a good idea *not* to hop in bed too swiftly. If we are like presents that we give to one another, make sure it takes some time for him to get that bow off. Put a few knots in it.

Now, if your religion, culture, or personal belief system advocates for no sex before marriage, it's important that you pick from the right dating pool. Find guys affiliated with your church, for example, who have the same views on sex.

Those are the extreme ends of the spectrum (fast and slow). Now let's look at the majority of people who fall somewhere in the middle. Patty Stanger, hostess of the TV show *Millionaire Matchmaker,* declares, "No sex until monogamy!" Honestly, I think that's a joke. Monogamy is ideal, but usually one person or the other wants to test the goods before making a commitment. In most cases, you're going to need to follow your heart and use your best judgment of when it makes sense for you to have sex with a new partner.

The main advice I can give you is to wait until you feel ready. Pressure is a really bad thing; if the guy's pressuring you, he's probably pressured other women and not that long ago. Women can be weak in a given moment with TDHAs—who seem to be able to take clothes off quicker than most. If he's really into you, he'll wait. Women tend to start bonding after having sex, in part because of the release of the hormone oxytocin. As such, it's wise to hold off until you feel safe and good about him. Let's say you jump into bed before you're ready and then find yourself getting attached quickly. If he jumps ship, you're going to feel crushed and taken advantage of.

That being said, all's fair in love and war and the effects of both can be devastating. There's no way to guarantee that your love won't go unreturned or that you won't experience heartbreak along the way. However, one way to maintain a degree of control over your love destiny is to stop yourself from having sex too soon. Think of it this way: If you had five dates with a guy you really liked and you only went as far as making out with him, you might feel really sad when he stops calling. But you would most likely feel much worse if you'd had sex with him.

The first heated moment might not come when you expect it. For that reason, keep condoms on hand. They're ready to go when you are. Along the same lines, invest in lingerie because you never know when the clothes are gonna come off!

Some of you might wait to have sex until the person has been tested for sexually transmitted diseases. I made Robert get tested before we slept together. Again, that is a personal decision. Either way, I would definitely advise you to use condoms until you know the guy is disease free and loyal to you only. If he's sleeping with other women, you are, too, in a sense. Always protect yourself. Don't fall for the guy's whimpers about hating condoms and how they just ruin the experience for him. Boohoo. Cry me a river, and go wrap that rascal! Furthermore, don't believe the stories that guys will tell you. He might say he just got tested a month ago and he's all set, but if any part of you thinks he's full of it, listen to that part of you! If you notice warts on his penis, don't let him convince you it's jockstrap irritation. Men can have an answer for everything. Always protect yourself.

When You're Rusty or Green (Or He Is)

If it's been a long time since you last had sex, you might feel like a guy's going to need a crowbar to get in there. And for those of you who are way out of practice, going to the ob-gyn doesn't count!

Women are often afraid of sex with a new person. Let's face it: You get on a roll with someone you've had sex with and you know how it works. It's like the fallback radio station that you can always turn to. You're comfortable with the music and don't have to change the dial. Your partner knows every bulge and scar on your body, everything you're afraid to unveil to a brand-new person. Then when you're single again, you find yourself reluctantly starting at square one. I don't care how in shape or good-looking you are, there are going to be physical imperfections that you're not comfortable with. And no, having sex in the dark is not the answer. Eventually the lights will come on.

I have my own story about this topic; I call it scar wars. As a result of having breast cancer, I had a mastectomy, which left behind scars. I was totally scared and upset about the idea of showing these scars to Robert, and he was aware that this was a hang-up for me. After about three months of dating, Robert booked us a hotel room in Nashville, where he had a work-related training. This was supposed to be the weekend of our first sexual encounter.

We were in the room and about to go out for lunch. Robert sat down on the bed, patted it, and said, "All right, let's get this scar-wars thing over with. I think you should just sit down and show me." I was taken aback. "Right now?" I said, "As if you're my doctor?" He said, "Yes, just like that." It was not a sexual space at all, just an icebreaker. I nervously took my top off and showed him. He said, "For God's sake, all that about that? What a beautiful body you have. You should be proud of it!" I put my clothes back on, we went out for lunch, and I never had a problem getting naked in front of him after that. And we did have our first sexual session that weekend!

Once you've had that first experience with a new person and you're thinking, wow, that was amazing, you aren't going to want to know why he is so good in bed. If he is, he's had a lot of experience. He didn't read it in a book or watch it on TV. He's been practicing and not with the same woman. One of my partners was a strapping, tall athlete who was unmarried many years of his life. Women wanted to sleep with him, and most of the time they got to. So, the truly talented are usually very seasoned! I suggest that you don't ask how they learned their lovemaking skills. The answer could ruin your post-coital bliss.

Now, whom would you rather have: The guy who's not that great in the sack but has everything you're looking for on your list? Or the guy who's exceptional in the bedroom but has very little else of what you want? I'll tell you whom you should choose: the guy with the list requirements.

First of all, there may be the guy who no matter what you say or do just has zero sexual intelligence, but most people can be made into better lovers if they're open to improvement. The guy who gets you all hot and bothered now will become a turn-off over time when he doesn't satisfy you in other ways. Women tend to go for the flashy guys. It's like the white elephant gift-exchange game. Everyone chooses the glitzy present with the pretty ribbons. The flashy males get chosen first because they stick out for their good looks (which usually leads to advanced sexual knowledge), but like the white elephant, you don't know what's going to be inside. There are a lot of wonderful guys who are just waiting to be discovered. If you find yourself with one, be patient.

He might not have a lot of experience or he could be nervous, but he probably wants to learn and improve. Wouldn't it be fun in dating if you came with instructions? You presented yourself with a card around your neck describing everything you love, and the guy provided a guide to everything that pleases him. Unfortunately it doesn't work that way, and you have to build a love life by communicating and demonstrating. Men like to know what the woman desires and vice versa.

A lot of men are open to women being playful and teaching them things. Sometimes men don't even know what they like. You know how sometimes you go to a restaurant and there are like ten items to choose from, and then other restaurants have pages and pages of menu options? Maybe this guy is pretty green and doesn't know that the pages-and-pages menu exists. If you're experienced and talented, present him with your big ol' repertoire and tell him to order up.

If you're not very experienced, there are plenty of ways to find inspiration. Whatever you do, I suggest taking baby steps in your quest for sexual excitement and improvement. You don't want to go from only trying one sexual position your whole life to attending a partner-swapping sex party. I think that sections of the *Kama Sutra,* an ancient Hindu text that covers lovemaking in great detail, are a good resource. There are a number of modern interpretations of the *Kama Sutra* that focus on how to kiss, embrace, set the mood, and try different positions. If you're a visual learner, I think you know where you can find inspiration!

Regardless of your experience levels, both partners in a monogamous relationship need to be clear about their wish lists (what they love to do or want to do). Everyone has their turn-ons and turn-offs, and some people are kinkier than others. Don't do anything that's going to unnerve you. People need to be good sexual matches in the sense that a really experimental guy is not going to end up satisfied by the woman who will only do two things in the bedroom: run and hide. It's really a simple conversation when you think about it. Talk about what you like, what you're willing to do, and what you're willing to consider. That talk evolves throughout your relationship as you grow to know each other more intimately.

No matter what you do, get a man who wants to be a pleaser, someone who's not always looking out for himself! Also, be able to laugh about sex, including during the act. Sex shouldn't be serious business, and it relieves some pressure to just find the humor in it and in each other.

Hot-and-Heavy Starts & Flameouts

Many relationships start hot and heavy and then slowly cool off. Others completely flame out to a point that the couples rarely get intimate and/ or end up sleeping in separate bedrooms. Let's take a look at why.

After the initial, potentially awkward first few sexual sessions, many couples have thriving sex lives for the first six to twelve months. Why? Because they don't have many responsibilities to each other. In the first few months, no one's talking about bills or taxes or how their twelve-year-old needs braces. It's all about wining and dining, having a good time, and getting physical. Everything is a beautiful conversation. Stage one is loving and lovemaking and getting to know each other in order to get to stage two.

When you're dating and not living with someone, you have a small window to be the best you can be, so it's easy to get your game face on. You could feel crappy all day, but all of a sudden it's seven o'clock, you shower and get ready, and you're the spontaneous, lively version of yourself. After being with your boyfriend, you can go home, flop on the bed, and put your old self back on. Most of us are pretty adept at being able to get in a good mood for a short portion of the day. As we spend more time with our partners, they see our crabbier sides and vice versa, and it all starts feeling a lot more real.

Once you're through the hot-and-heavy beginning, responsibility starts to get in the way. You have to deal with things that don't make you feel sexy, like mortgage payments and sick children—especially when you're married. I find that couples who stop having sex often have allowed too many responsibilities, excuses, and time to get in the way. We are all creatures of habit, and not having sex, just like anything else, can become a habit.

Financial worries can really hurt the sex life: *How are we going to pay the bills? We might lose the house. We're both working two jobs and hanging on by a thread. We've got kids to put to bed and mouths to feed.* I can appreciate all of those concerns. Sometime before the day is up, though, you've got to take a moment to connect. I don't care if it only lasts five minutes or it's a simple statement like, "Honey, I love you. I know you've had a hard day." It's a small gesture, but it's a building block. Those little moments of love and care build to something; a couple might not have had sex for six months, but all of a sudden after this extended period of being supportive and kind to each other, they'll make love. It will seem like it came out of nowhere, but it didn't. The love needed to manifest itself.

There's too much focus on the word "sex." Affection is what matters. Do you still have affection for each other? That's how you maintain and rekindle intimacy. You have to feel celebrated by the love of your life. It's like the person who lives right by the beach and doesn't even look out the window anymore to admire the ocean view. Couples get caught up without seeing, feeling, or appreciating each other. They become calloused; once they've dropped the slack, they don't pick it up again to create romance. It's very important to be loving and affectionate to your partner.

Sex lives can stay fiery or go in the tank, and a lot of it depends on respect. People don't want to have sex with a partner whom they don't respect. I had a fantastic sex life with one of my husbands until our marital issues became overwhelming, and I lost so much respect for him that the sexual part just died for me. You can dig and dig and dig, but when you've stopped respecting someone, it's hard to get the fire back. Then too much time goes by and you can't get it back at all. Respect gets lost over money, infidelity, parenting decisions, addiction, and overall bad behavior.

Sex is as much a mental connection as it is a physical one—unless you're a porn star. Be aware of the mental connection you have with your partner because when it slips, your sex life usually does too. And when that mental connection is strong, so usually is your sex life.

Another observation I've made is that mental exhaustion is far more tiring than physical exhaustion when it comes to sex. For example, if you're dating the owner of a small company who has to make difficult financial and operational decisions on a frequent basis, he'll often return home at the end of the day completely drained. To get him out of that stressful, exhausted headspace and thinking about sex is very challenging. On the flipside, I don't know a construction worker or physical laborer who's not great in bed. He may have worked his butt off carrying wood on his shoulders or digging a coalmine, but Mr. Physical Labor has the reputation of a bedroom star. I think it's because the physical guy doesn't have to think as much as the mental guy in order to do his job well. Then at the end of the day, the physical guy sees sex with you as just the next physical task that he has to do, while the mental guy needs to stop ruminating over the financial statements or product launch.

An affluent doctor (who became my client after his divorce) had been building his practice and was consumed by his work. He and his wife were in the process of renovating their home in Rancho Santa Fe, a very wealthy town, when she left him a note saying she was running off with the contractor. Why? The contractor was around to have sex with her, and she fell in love with all the attention she was getting. Women want attention over money. Attention is number one. The guy who gives a woman attention is going to win every time—until he runs out of money!

Beyond the Word "Sex"

To me, sex doesn't necessarily mean going the whole enchilada. I really refrain from thinking that sex only means intercourse. It is a playful act and can be a lot of kissing and hugging or your partner coming up from behind you and kissing the back of your neck. Sex can even be a feeling of excitement that you get when you make eye contact with someone you find attractive. I think that people put too much emphasis on the actual act of one body being inside another body, and that's why the pharmaceutical industry makes huge profits selling Cialis and Viagra. People think they're failing if they're not penetrating, and that's really not true. In a healthy relationship, warmth and attention need to be present to have a good sex life. Whatever follows from there is the crescendo.

The desire and care we feel for another person keeps us happy and vibrant. Did you know that a hug has the ability to lower blood pressure and ease stress, as well as bonding you to your partner? You can have that kind of special intimacy at any age, and it doesn't require acrobatic love-making to accomplish. When that feeling isn't there, it's a sign that the relationship is pulling apart.

How Often Should We Do the Deed?

Sexual frequency varies a lot from couple to couple. How often should people have sex? To me, it's whatever works for the couple, whether it's once a week or more or less. I know some readers are going to want a direct answer from me, so when put on the spot, I'd say twice a week for the full-on act is a good target.

Let's say a couple goes to Tahiti and has sex every day twice a day because it just feels right. They're in bathing suits with easy access and no responsibilities to run off to. Real life is different. Jobs, kids, etc., get in the way. I don't believe that people should make frequency demands of their partners as in, "We must have sex three times a week." The timing needs to feel natural, not forced. In long-term relationships, there can be pressure to suddenly make sex happen, like you're filling a mandatory quota. If you release that pressure and let things flow, it's going to happen. Sex is generated by attention. Two people who work on giving each other attention and saying positive things to each other build a platform for a sexual act.

But if a husband talks disrespectfully to his wife throughout the week, and it's Saturday night and he's like, okay, we need to have sex, her response (whether she says it aloud or just brushes him off) is going to be, "No, we don't. You've been treating me disrespectfully. Why all of a sudden am I supposed to be this hot woman in the bedroom when I have felt picked on all week?"

It works the other way around, too. Women can snuff out the mood by nagging or criticizing their male partners. Whenever the week starts going in a bad direction as far as his and your behavior is concerned, you have to ask yourself: Would I want to sleep with him now? Or, would he want to sleep with me? If your answer is no, then say your sincere "honey, I love you" and initiate a caring interaction. Always create the right stage for your relationship to blossom; true affection and enjoyable sex are not going to happen otherwise. One partner might go through with the act without being into it, which can lead to more resistance down the line and more sexual dissatisfaction.

If the respect is strong in a relationship, but one person wants to have sex more often than the other, together they're going to have to reach a compromise. Again, men are creatures of habit. Occasionally, then, you have to put a general maximum in place that they agree is acceptable and can work with. One of my husbands was a hot-blooded romantic fool and wanted to have sex every day. Sex was like eating to him—a daily habit. After the initial honeymoon phase of the relationship, I had to set new parameters because sex every day was not going to work for me. In my opinion, if you do anything every day it loses its charm. Eating lobster is a treat, but eating it every night is not. I personally think it's the same with lovemaking.

If you find yourself in a situation where your partner wants more sex than feels right to your appetite, you have to be very thoughtful about the way you approach the subject. You could say that you regard lovemaking with him to be special and you want it to stay that way, but if the expectation becomes that sex needs to happen every day it's going to lose its charm. You want to look forward to it, not make it a daily must like brushing your teeth. He might not be thrilled by your message, but it's much better to explain yourself than to keep turning him down, which will lead to frustration and conflict.

Whatever you do, don't use sex as a reward/punishment system. You want him to know that you enjoy sex, and it's not something he gets when he's good and doesn't get when he's bad. That's a situation ripe for disaster! Of course, if your appetite is stronger than his, you've got to be understanding and willing to compromise if you want the relationship to work.

Spontaneity and Foreplay

A good sex life is spontaneous. When you are affectionate with your partner on an ongoing basis, you build an undercurrent of attraction and tension. As a result, you don't know when or where sex is going to happen, which makes for an exciting sex life. I mean you can plan for it in the sense that you could schedule a romantic evening and know that the night's events will lead to an intimate moment, but I don't suggest saying, "Let's have sex on Sunday morning." It shouldn't be a chore or obligation, and you want sex to happen when you both feel the desire for it.

In addition to spontaneity, foreplay is extremely important! Most women want a man who takes her face and spends time kissing her—soft and sweet and gentle—and knows how to love her through her lips. I had a husband who didn't like a lot of foreplay, so I had to work with him on that because the kissing and affectionate touching of foreplay is a big part of the sexual process. In fact, as you get older, if foreplay is all you have in the end, then that's still terrific because that satisfaction can last forever.

Generally speaking, women like tenderness and lots of foreplay, while men are ready to lunge into the act, swords at the ready. Guys are looking at the clock and want to get it all in—bundle it like a cable company. Women want things done slowly; they want men to take their time with them. Since women crave the buildup, but men's one-track minds have them focused on the end game, the contradictory priorities can cause problems. After too many sessions without enough foreplay, women start to turn down men's advances. They're getting fit into the guy's schedule and not liking the wham bam, thank you ma'am arrangement. Or women are dissatisfied and faking orgasms in order to make the guy think he's top banana.

In my matchmaking and relationship coaching, a lack of foreplay is one of the biggest sexual complaints I hear from women. For a woman I think the perfect amount of time for sex is one hour. It's enough time for the couple to hug and kiss and hold each other and talk afterwards. Tell and show your man how to slow down and how you like to be touched. Communication about sexual needs and wants is absolutely crucial to a couple's happy intimacy. If you feel like everything is a quickie and that's not working for you, pretty soon you're going to avoid having sex, which isn't good for either of you. Some of you might have to teach your guy how to kiss well. You want him to ease up on the hard kisses and keep that tongue from going crazy. Gross! We're all works in progress, so allow him to teach you some things too!

Sex Through the Ages

Women in early adulthood have beautifully-moist reproductive skin because their hormones are raging. When you're young, kissing and touching can make you all juicy and wonderful so that all that stands between you and sex are your clothes. You don't get to be as spontaneous starting around age fifty. You're no longer at a point where your body is always ready, as it is in your youth, which means you have to prepare more. If your body's not producing enough juice, it could be time to buy vaginal moisturizers and lube.

As you go through menopause, you get dry from lack of hormones and are unsure how anything is going to make it in there. Your vaginal lining also thins. For some women, at this time having sex becomes very painful, which is why various products exist. There are injectable creams; I call them creams for the crotch. The effect of the cream doesn't last long, so you're not hoping for a long session! Men might need a little help from their friends as well. I call Cialis and Viagra the weekend warriors—take a pill and be ready for action for three days. Well, the industry hasn't come up with a pill for a woman that keeps her lubricated for three days. That's what women really need—instant moisture that lasts!

Though I'd say in general that your overall sex drive drops as you get older, I think it's all about your attitude. Believe it or not, people can still have sex in their eighties and beyond. Keep in mind that "sex" doesn't have to be penetration; there are a lot of ways to achieve sexual gratification. And if being romantic and loving with each other with kisses and hugs is all the couple wants to do at ninety years old, good for them! That's a happy sex life! Now let's take a look at how you figure out whether the sex and other aspects of your relationship are good enough to move forward together.

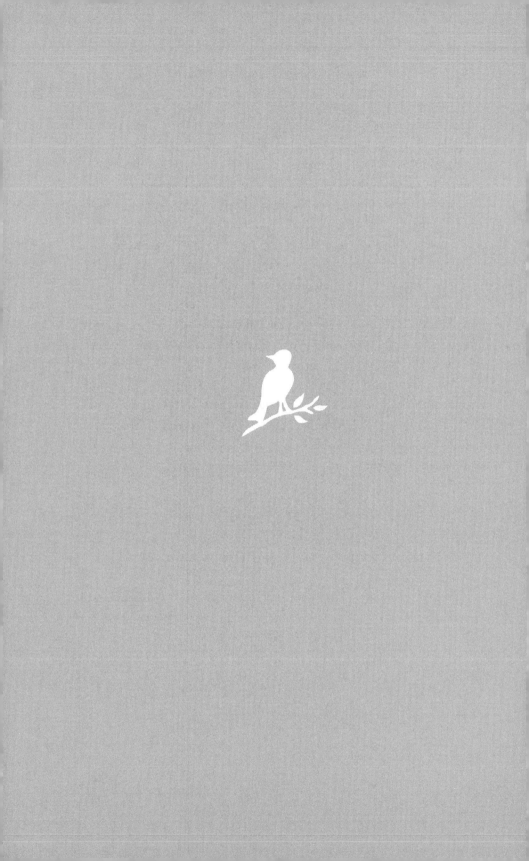

Forward or Not? You Can't Change That

IF YOU'VE BEEN DATING THE SAME GUY for three or four months, it's time to decide whether to move forward with him. Dating is a bit like fishing. It's catch and release. Sometimes you reel in a keeper, and sometimes you need to throw a puny one back in the water to grow up or swim another day.

A Reason, a Season, or a Lifetime

The people who enter our lives fall into one of those three categories. Let's say you date a guy for a few months who inspires you to go back to school and finish your degree. The relationship doesn't end up lasting for long, but he brought that very important motivation into your life. He's an example of a "reason."

In your early twenties, maybe you had a two-year relationship with a chef. You lived in New York, had an exciting time together, but you drifted apart. You wanted to move back to San Francisco, and he got a job offer in Paris. Au revoir! He was a "season" guy, and you will look back fondly on those years after enough time has passed.

And then there is the lifetime guy. He is the one with whom you will see out the rest of your days. My first three husbands were seasons; I really believe Robert is the lifetime. Some of you are saying, "Sure, Barbara. I'm not holding my breath!" Well, he is closer to death than the other three, which increases his chances. Kidding aside, the reason why I believe he'll be the lifetime guy is he shows me on a daily basis how much he loves me on many levels.

Now, after the first three or four months of dating, it's important not to force a guy into the lifetime role when he isn't a good long-term match. Let's face it—women tend to hold on when what they really should do is let go. He's fun and sweet, but he's not enough of a go-getter for you, so you don't picture it working. Accept that you've had a good time for a few months; maybe he taught you about astronomy or guitar or flipping omelets. Take the good with the bad—it's all a learning experience—and find your next adventure. Free him up to find a better match. You never want to waste your time or his on a bad match or a dead end. Women desperately try to fit the proverbial square peg in a round hole, and they keep coming up with lame reasons why the guy's worth keeping. Use your emotional energy and time in a more productive way.

When you're first dating someone, picture your future like a movie. Do you see the two of you playing out in a fantastic way up on the big screen? Would it be an entertaining and heartwarming film? Whether it's kids you want or to travel across the world, do you see it happening with this person? You both need to visualize where the story could take you and like where the plot is headed.

Along the same lines, if the life you've lived thus far could play out in front of you and entertain you, then you've lived a good life. Maybe the story even makes you blush at times. The colorful parts of our lives—the ups, the downs, the why-did-I-do-that moments—make for a good movie. Watching a film about someone who lived in the same house, had the same job, and pursued the same hobbies for thirty years would be boring. If you think you've been stuck and don't like what you see, don't wallow in regret. Make changes. Jump back into life. Furthermore, don't be afraid of your plotlines unfolding in a way you didn't expect. If you thought this guy had potential, but now after three months of dating you don't see it, oh well. Next!

Recheck the Dream Match List and Your Pulse

The first thing you should do after several months of dating is to grab the Dream Match List you made and recheck it carefully. Is the guy still meeting those must-have requirements? He led you to believe that he was financially stable, but he's asked you twice to loan him fifty dollars. You don't have to be a genius to figure out that his bank account does not look anything like Warren Buffett's. Don't make excuses for him; see the picture for what it is.

It's possible that a couple of wish-list items won't stay in place and that you may have to tweak a few habits and lifestyles to make it work. As long as that's okay with both of you, super. But if he's not meeting your basic requirements, he should be toast. Wash that man right out of your hair.

You also have to ask yourself: Is the excitement still there? At first he wooed you with nice dinners and a weekend getaway, but by the end of the fourth month, going out has been replaced by watching Padres games on the couch. You're getting bored, and he's not putting energy into your relationship. The first few months of a relationship should be dazzling, so if it's already dull, do yourself a favor and pull the plug.

Is he spending enough time with you? If you're still just seeing him once a week and you'd like it to be more, that's not a good sign. When he doesn't want to commit too much of his time to you, that means you're not a priority. Maybe he doesn't want anything serious, or maybe he's just not serious about you. It could be that he's very busy with work and his children from a prior marriage. If that's the case, are you okay being with a guy who just can't find time for you? When you don't want to spend much time with him, that's also a sign to walk on.

You Can't Change That

Several months into dating it's common to say to yourself, "I don't like how he (fill in the blank), but I think I can change that." No, my dear, you probably cannot.

When I first started dating Robert I thought I could get him to slim down by fifteen pounds. After taking his wine away, I decided the calorie reduction just wasn't worth his uptight and crabby behavior. I am joking, but in all seriousness, hoping someone will change in a significant way is unrealistic. Though we are all works in progress, we can't sculpt a perfect partner. If there's a trait you dislike initially in him, like laziness, don't start telling yourself that you're going to change him because you're not! Most women think they can get a man to change. We're glass-half-full types when it comes to love. We think we can influence a guy by inserting our suggestions and wishes on him. He often thinks he's fine just the way he is, thank you very much.

It's possible that he will be willing to change some small habits, but don't assume that he'll just roll over like a dog, let you rearrange his life, and wag his tail as you do it. Let's say it drives you nuts that he leaves his clothes on the floor when he stays at your place and that he smokes cigars nightly—the smell of which make you gag. You need to nicely express that those habits aren't working for you. If he changes voluntarily without resentment and keeps the change up without a bunch of nagging from you, then that's a thumbs-up. But maybe he just does the quick fix Band-Aid trick, picking up his cigar-smelly clothes one day and the next day leaving them strewn on the carpet. Annoying!

If you find yourself nitpicking him within the first three months, stop doing it and break up with him. The first phase should be happy and fun; overall, the relationship should be flowing along contentedly with minimal drama. If it isn't, something's wrong and it's time to move on. When you want to change the car he drives, the way he talks to people, and his career, then he is not the guy for you. It's the golden rule you learned in kindergarten, along with how to tie your shoes: treat others how you would like to be treated. And for goodness sake, don't waste time on a bad match! Next!

The People Who Scrap It Too Quickly

More often than not, women hold on to a relationship for way too long, but other women don't hold on long enough in the beginning. Because there are many people out there to possibly connect with, some single folks are prompted to "sample" without ever sticking with the same person. I think of dating like dieting (even though I don't like that word) in that people give up too quickly. You think a guy is a good fit. Then four months later, a few annoyances arise, and you want to scrap the whole thing. It's like giving up the nutritional plan and going for the candy bar. Let's face it: It's easier to be single, to not share, to not try. Just in the way it's easier to eat whatever we want and pack on the pounds again.

Certain individuals have a hard time transitioning from the first few dates into the real life of grocery shopping and upset stomachs. As soon as it gets real, they lose interest. If you tend to throw guys onto the scrap heap before you've given them a chance, think about what's compelling you to do that. You might be trying to protect yourself. But you need to decide if you like living that way. By throwing up walls, you can find yourself in a lonely place. If this is you, try giving your relationships more of a chance in the beginning.

First-Phase Test

At the three- or four-month marker, you need clarity. I don't want you wasting your time, so ask yourself the following questions before deciding whether you're moving forward with or without him. (These questions, with spaces for your responses, are provided in the back of the book on page 194. If you've been dating someone for a few months now, please take this First-Phase Test after reading this chapter. It'll help you figure out whether he qualifies for the next round!)

1. How do you feel?

How do you know if someone is good for you? Pay attention to how you feel at the end of the day. If your partner has been making cracks about your weight or intelligence, you're not going to feel attractive or smart. Does he say things like, "Don't you have any other jeans you can wear?" or "I thought you said you could cook; this is gross"? Too many women suffer from low self-esteem and think they deserve to be put down. They don't! Don't ever stay with a guy who makes you feel bad about yourself!

In a good relationship, people are encouraged and adored. Your partner should celebrate you and love you for who you are. We need to feel admired as a whole person, not judged and analyzed by our parts. When you're not feeling good in a relationship, you need to figure out why. Is it something he's doing or saying? Are you not excited about him? How is he with you when you're down? When you're sick?

The first few months of a relationship should, for the most part, go swimmingly, so if they aren't, don't stick around to watch the relationship drown. Move on.

2. Are your active/inactive levels balanced?

The amount of time you spend resting and playing should be compatible with his. If your perfect Sunday is hiking, doing yoga, and taking mini road trips, and his is watching DVDs and drinking beer on the porch, you're probably not a good match. You can't have one person saying, "come on already," while the other is like, "relax already. Why don't you just sit down and chill out?"

I'm a busy, on-the-go person, but I once dated a tennis pro who I couldn't keep up with. Because I was losing weight and wearing myself out, I faced the fact that we weren't well matched and stopped seeing him. You shouldn't find yourself constantly frustrated, bored, wishing you could do something, or wishing you could just take it easy. As more time goes on, your partner becomes like an adult playmate, so you want to choose one with similar interests and energy levels.

3. Does he handle money well and is he generous with it?

He says he'd love to take you out to dinner, but the rent is due so it's instant ramen time. You have to take money matters very seriously! Disagreements over finances have doomed many a marriage. Pick up information about his financial situation by being observant. Maybe he makes a lot of money but blows it foolishly. Or he's El Cheapo who only takes you out during happy hour. If simple observation of his habits isn't revealing enough, find indirect ways of getting intel. When he treats you to dinner on his American Express card, for example, you could say that Am Ex is your card of choice, though the rewards have been a little lackluster lately. If he says, "That's the least of my worries. I can barely keep up with the minimum, and this card is almost at the limit," then you might be maxed out on him.

Perhaps you have financial problems, and we all know that misery loves company. You're broke; he's broke. Maybe you can help each other move forward. But maybe you'll be a mutually horrible influence. Personal finance is not an area that deserves the benefit of the doubt. Look for the red flags and get out of the way before the oncoming train of foreclosure, debt, gambling problems, etc., runs you over.

Secondly, has he made any attempt to buy you anything? I don't care if it's shampoo. When you're at the grocery-store checkout counter, does he just stand there and let you pay, or does he open his wallet? Is he treating for dinners and movies? Again, it's not the amount of money that counts; it's whether he's generous with what he has. The Mr.-Even-Steven type who hasn't even bought you a beverage has got to go. You want a guy who is thoughtful and generous with the resources he has. The attitude he holds now toward money will carry on over time, so be honest with yourself as to whether it's working for you. Don't expect his financial situation or tendencies around money to change.

4. Are your diet and daily habits an easy match?

He's a meat-and-potatoes guy and you're a vegetarian. He thinks your health food sucks. You're grossed out by his bloody steak. How is this going to work? Sometimes people have flexibility with their eating habits and can make simple compromises. Other times it's oil and water, no pun intended. And it's not just about food. You're a goody two shoes who has no more than two drinks a week, but he drinks three martinis every night and smokes two packs a day. Extremes don't work because no one can fit into the other person's world when there are such great differences. Take a look at your diets, sleeping patterns (i.e., things like morning person, night owl), exercise levels, and other daily habits to see how well they're mixing together.

I know many women who have been single for a long time and are so incredibly uptight about what they must eat and do every day that they are nearly impossible to match up. They're not enjoyable to go out to dinner with because they're always telling the waitress that they're gluten-free, can't have dairy or MSG, and that they'll only eat locally-grown salad greens. And the guy is slinking down in his chair thinking, uh-oh, even ordering food is a total production with her. High-maintenance, finicky people are not fun. Their obsessions have gotten in the way of making simple daily-life transactions. The drop-dead-gorgeous woman who is ridiculously fussy will start to lose her sex appeal when the guy finds her so over the top that he can barely stand her company.

Everyone wants to enjoy life and have a few laughs, especially guys. If you want to keep a guy in your life, don't be a finicky pain in the neck who won't go out in the rain because your hair will frizz and needs an hour to get ready just to walk the beach. I know a guy who broke up with a woman because she had to run six miles every day. As a couple, their plans had to work around her jogging requirement. "We can't go to that barbecue at two o'clock, because I won't be back in time from my run to shower and get ready." Rules that work for you as a single person might not work in a relationship. Rigor mortis will set in when you're dead; don't let it happen while you're living!

5. Do you complement/complete each other?

Everyone is looking for something they lack. What you bring to the table, such as a can-do attitude, can be just what the other person feels he's missing. You can empower others by being a good influence. Robert drank Pepsi and ate cream sauces and other fattening foods before we met. He was looking for someone to lead the way in the health department, and I was a good fit. Noticing the way I ran my business, he saw financial fixer-upper all over me and helped me trim my excess spending.

Two people in a relationship should complement each other well, filling in where the other leaves off.

I find that men are fixers. They like their tools. In the early stage of a relationship, they're thinking: What does she need fixed? She loves animals but lives in a small apartment. I have a huge yard where her dog could run around. Men like to feel useful and at times heroic, but don't confuse that with neediness. Men do not like needy women! They want a strong woman who also makes them feel like they have a helpful role to play. If men don't see how they could be beneficial to a woman in some way, they get intimidated. But they don't want a basket case.

Though it's common for opposites to attract, the only way that works is when you respect what is different about the other person. Let's say you're a brainy, quiet person who makes a living as an engineer, and you start dating a guy who is a vivacious personal trainer. As long as you respect his personality and occupation and enjoy what he contributes to your life and vice versa, it can work. But if you're the breadwinner and homeowner and he lives paycheck to paycheck, and that drives you crazy, you'll both become unhappy. Make sure the two of you find the relationship mutually beneficial and are grateful to each other for the unique gifts and qualities you both bring to the table.

6. How is his temperament?

Does he get snappy with the valet guy or rude to the bartender out of the blue? Abrupt flare-ups are a red flag! Has he gotten angry with you? Possessive? On the other extreme, if he's real mellow, does that work for you? You like to take the stage and he's background music. Maybe that's perfect because he doesn't draw attention away from you, but maybe it doesn't work because he's not enough of a standout. You want your temperaments to be compatible. Usually two intense people don't match well because they burn each other out; there's no one to lighten the mood. Know yourself and your needs and see if his temperament works well with yours.

On any meds? This might seem strange to you, but you wouldn't want to get nine months into a relationship and then discover that a person has bipolar disorder and is on medication for it. You don't want to give out too much information about yourself at first, and that obviously works the other way around; however, you don't want to miss something major by the end of the three-month marker!

You should be aware of the person's health issues and whether he is receiving any kind of treatment. Let's say you take sleeping pills when you have problems with insomnia. You might share that with him and then ask, "Do you take anything that keeps you together?" Based on his answer and the way he handles himself, you need to decide whether this works for you. We all have problems—that's for sure! I just find that people minimize serious considerations because they want so badly for the relationship to work. You have to be willing to accept the worst-case scenarios that the health issue could bring about and not put a Pollyanna spin on reality. Don't assume he'll get better because he's with you.

Aside from doctor's prescriptions, you definitely want to look at the amount of over-the-counter goodies he ingests. Is he a big drinker or smoker or pain-pill popper? Be very leery about moving forward with him if you see any signs of substance abuse.

7. Is he a good sexual match?

One person can't be a bunny rabbit, while the other could take it or leave it. As I explained in chapter seven, sex should be a celebration, not a feeling of oh, no, he wants that again. On the flipside, if you think he has a low libido and you want more bedroom time and are constantly frustrated, this is not going to work. You can always try to compromise, but in situations where people's drives are opposite of each other, it's hard to find an agreeable happy medium. While it is common for couples to start off hot and heavy, it's never good to assume that anyone's overall sex drive will drop or increase. If the sex is good, make sure that's not the only asset keeping you in the relationship. There should be a lot of other factors, too, like his intelligence, kindness, faith in God, or whatever you're looking for on your list. If those factors are in place, but he's not terribly impressive in the bedroom, see if he's open to improvement and can learn new tricks.

8. Does he have the gift of gab?

Do you have good conversations? Is he too quiet for you? Too chatty for you? Do you feel like he gets what you're trying to say and has thoughtful responses? Does he listen to you? Oral communication is crucial to the health of a relationship. He could be the hottest drummer who ever graced the planet, but if he can't express himself in anything other than four-word sentences, then you're going to get tired of trying to read his mind. Now, some people are quiet and don't like a lot of talking. That's fine—whatever works for you.

I personally can't stand lulls in a conversation. I remember walking to a beachfront restaurant with my then-husband. He didn't say a word. During dinner he barely talked. Finally I said, "Don't you want to talk to me?" He said, "No, let's just be quiet with ourselves and enjoy our food." I knew that was a sign that our relationship was falling apart. Along the same lines, however, I need quiet time every day, which means it's important for me to be with someone who understands and allows that.

When women babble about a lot of nothing, men find the conversation frivolous and tune out. Ask yourself if you're talking volumes without actually saying anything. If so, that's a habit to work on.

9. What are his friends like?

How many close friends does he have? What are they like? You don't want the guy who never socializes with friends or family members, because he will not have a world outside yours. You will feel suffocated when he's calling you eleven times a day and following you around like a shadow, or feel bored when he has very little to say and doesn't want to spend a lot of time with you, either. Loners don't make good partners because often they're either controlling or very withdrawn.

On the other hand, the guy who likes to have a lot of male-bonding time, let's say, playing sports and going out drinking with the guys, tends to be the player type who likes his freedom. He wants to grab you off the shelf when it's convenient and doesn't want you to complain that he doesn't spend enough time with you. Unless you want to be Little-Miss-Wait-by-the-Phone, I suggest you move on. It's important that in general you like his friends and vice versa. If you have incompatible friend groups, that is going to put a strain on your social life and, by extension, your relationship.

Our friends allow us to take the past with us. They represent where we've been during various stages of time. Seeing and interacting with your new partner's friends will provide you with a collage of his life and reveal a lot about who he's been and is.

10. For single parents, does he pass the kid test?

Don't introduce your children to your boyfriend unless you're very happy with him, hope that the relationship lasts, and believe that it will. Give it at least three months. You don't want your children to experience men coming in and out of your life or theirs. It's not fair, and it's confusing. If he passes the three-month test and you're ready to introduce him, pay attention to your children's reactions. Unlike adults, kids don't sugarcoat things. If your six-year-old says he's boring, think about that. Is it because he is boring in general or doesn't relate well to children? Observe how the guy behaves around your kids—like a natural dad? Nervous but trying? With disdain, as though your children are leeches? (I'll discuss this subject more in chapters nine and twelve.)

11. How is he while out of his element?

When you're dating and trying to figure out how compatible you are with a guy, I highly recommend you have an experience with him out of his normal element. You could go camping, take a weekend trip to wine country, or whatever fits both of your budgets and tastes. You have to shake things up to see how the other person deals with out-of-the-ordinary situations. I believe that you don't really know a guy until you've gone on a trip with him.

However, make sure the guy initiates the first trip. It's a test of his organizational skills and how interested he is in you. If you plan the first weekend getaway and book the hotel, then you've taken his power away and also set a precedent that you will be the one to plan vacations and special weekends. Unless you're really into control, I suggest not taking sole ownership of the event-planner role.

While away, you will see parts of your partner that you may not have noticed. Pay attention to how he reacts to new situations and how well you're getting along. A different environment can strengthen your romance or expose deep cracks.

I knew a guy who decided to take his love interest on a luxurious trip to Europe after they had dated for about a month. She's a bombshell workout freak, and he was exceedingly proud of her appearance. They flew first class to Paris and stayed in a swanky hotel. He has a passion for art and history and wanted to go to museums, but she was completely uninterested and instead wanted to shop at places like Louis Vuitton and Chanel. The vast difference in travel preferences caused friction, and they started fighting.

One night they were strolling around Paris within view of the Eiffel Tower. It started to rain, so he opened up a big umbrella and reached out to draw her under it. He thought, what a quintessential romantic evening— we're in Paris in the rain staring at the shimmering lights of the Eiffel Tower. She ruptured his fantasy when she snapped, "Stop trying to control me!" He was so shocked and upset that he shoved the umbrella into her hand and stormed off. They flew back to the States in separate rows of the plane and never went out again. Twenty-five thousand dollars later, he discovered in a very disappointing way that this relationship was not going to last. All the more reason that the first trip should be on a modest scale!

12. Are your future goals aligned?

I'll cover this in more depth next chapter, but for now ask yourself if you want the same things in the future: Marriage? Children? A house in the country? An apartment in the city? A life of travel and volunteer work? If you really want children, for example, and he never does, it does not make sense to continue dating.

Before I set you loose to answer those twelve questions, let's infiltrate the male camp for a moment.

Are You Passing His Bar?

What are men looking for at the three- or four-month marker? One consideration is how willing the woman is to hook up or have sex (which you may or may not have gotten to at this point—remember it's totally up to you!). Whether or not it's not the whole enchilada, does she shrug off advances and say she has a headache, or is she showing that she's physically attracted to him? Men are also questioning whether she has a sense of humor and is fun. Some men will want to see that women can make social plans without going overboard and plotting out their entire month. Guys don't want to constantly have the conversation of "What are we going to do tonight?" "I don't know. What do you want to do tonight?" That's going to get dull. At the same time, though, men want to make sure that women haven't infringed on their male-bonding or solo time.

Another checklist item that men consider is this: Has she been true to who she was in the very beginning of the relationship? There are women who pretend to be active and easygoing, and then as time passes their true colors come out. A guy might think, we went out a lot in the first month and now she's often tired on Saturday night and just wants to watch TV. Or, she was totally cool about me hanging out with my guy friends on Sundays to watch football and now she whines about it.

Men start to see patterns and then evaluate whether those patterns work for them. For example, if the woman is a finicky, high-maintenance health nut who's popping every vitamin known to man and then is always complaining that something's wrong—she's quite a hypochondriac—the guy is going to wonder whether this is someone he wants to be around. Many women are drawn to drama and seem to cause it wherever they go, and he's getting tired of that, too. "Why can't she just get along with my buddy's girlfriend? Now she doesn't want us to get together as couples with them anymore." Try to get perspective on your own behavior to see if you're being enjoyable, reasonable, and loving. You might have work to do!

The main point of this chapter is to get you to think about whether this is a person you should continue dating. If it's a fling with no long-term potential, let go now. The longer that women stay in relationships, the harder it is for them to end them. Don't allow time to become your enemy because you weren't willing to make informed decisions early on. You are a time dominatrix. Allow no weak men to get past you!

For those of you finding yourselves at the end of that critical first phase of dating, the three- or four-month mark, it's time to take the test on page 194. Keep in mind that your guy should measure up well on each question. A tiny hesitation here and an iffy result there might not doom your forward progress, but anything worse than that is bye-bye time.

Keeping the Eye on the Prize: Planning, Fighting, Testing

AFTER SEVERAL MONTHS OF DATING, you get into real life. You're spending a lot of time together and there isn't the formality of "Is it okay if I come over?" The nervous politeness dissipates, and you can be much more relaxed in who you are. You've put down the script and stopped trying to be perfect. He's seen you without your makeup on; you've watched him suffer through the flu. You're not flipping pancakes every morning with an ear-to-ear grin on your face.

Reality and responsibility start to set in and you experience each other's grumpy, sad, and pleasant moments. You'll fight; you'll see some red flags; you'll evaluate how day-to-day life is treating you. You'll also start thinking more and more about where the relationship is headed and figuring out whether to stay or go.

The Plan and the Ticking Clock

A friend of mine named Michelle believes, "Women should have a plan. They should know what they want. If he fits in your plan, super. But don't just settle for his plan or be on his time frame." I completely agree. What do you want for your own future?

In your early twenties, I think you should play the field. After twenty-five, most women are ready to get at least a little more serious. A twenty-six-year-old woman, for instance, might decide that she wants two children by the time she's thirty. If that's the case, she better figure out whether her current boyfriend is a keeper. If he doesn't want kids, she needs to release him so she can find a better match.

You don't want time to just go by, because it will! You can be with someone and blink and two years will have passed. And as time passes, so do certain opportunities. Very early on in the relationship, two people need to talk about what they want out of life and how they plan to pursue it. Certainly by the end of three months, you should have a very good sense of the other person's goals and intended life path. I suggest you start the dialogue earlier than that. He plans to live on a ranch in Montana and have five children. You prefer Manhattan and want one child. How is this ever going to work?

By sharing your hopes and dreams, you're not telling your new love interest that he has to spend the rest of his life with you. You're just finding out if it looks like you have compatible goals. If a thirty-one-year-old woman really wants to travel the world, when the guy tells her on the second date that he has never left Idaho and never plans to, she should enjoy the rest of the date and cross him off her list of eligible bachelors. Next up!

For relationships to survive, people's future visions need to align. Otherwise, one or both partners will feel unfulfilled, and resentment will build. That's not to say that compromises don't work, but those compromises should be relatively easy to make and not require that anyone give up too much.

If marriage and children are a priority to you, find out early on if he wants to get married at some point in the future, how he feels about having children, and what time frame he has in mind. If your vision of marriage and family does not resemble his (he's like, "Why get married? It's just a piece of paper," but you want the big wedding, the ring, and the honeymoon), move on. Breakups get harder and harder as time goes by. Don't spin your wheels. And it's not just marriage and family that you should ask about. It's career and education choices, travel plans, and so forth. If you're in your sixties, it's the retirement plan. Whatever your age, stage, or style, find out if he looks like a good fit for you.

By the six-month marker, you should definitely have a handle on how well real life is working out with this person. If it's good and the future looks promising, at the end of a year you'll be sinking or swimming. The hot romance might start fizzling as small habits drive you crazy, or maybe you'll still be thrilled about this guy.

By one and a half years of dating, you should be engaged. Once engaged, I think couples should move in together, but not before. *By two and a half years of dating, you should be married.* Why? Because you don't want to end up feeling stuck and without momentum. *The idea of marriage starts to fade out if a couple stays together too long without being engaged.* The guy thinks, why fix or change things? He's happy or, at the very least, not put in a position of feeling scared. He doesn't have pressure and he has you. Believe me, if you want more, you're not going to feel satisfied. You'll see your friends getting married and having children. You'll attend countless showers and wonder why you're not celebrating any milestones.

After two years with no major commitment, people (especially women) in relationships can start to get bored. They want that freshness back or to go on to the next step. Everyone would like to repeat the beginning of a relationship because that's when the romance is at its peak. Those are the magical years that we see playing up on the big screen. So if that time passes and there is no engagement (a step that brings the excitement back into the relationship and reminds us of its beginning), the relationship stagnates, and the couple can get in the doldrums, which then makes commitment harder to come by. When that happens, the couple questions whether there's something wrong with the relationship when the problem is often the lack of momentum. There's a sense of "this isn't going anywhere."

Generally, women want the feeling of moving forward—of consistently creating and building a future with a significant other. Only the relationships that stay in motion will thrive. Motion meaning always having a plan, whether it's planning trips, a wedding, a dinner party, how many kids you're going to have, or what you're going to do in retirement.

When the motion stops, people get stuck. And being stuck sucks! We'll look at engagement and marriage much more closely in upcoming chapters, but for now I just want you having an idea of the big-picture plan.

Daily Lives in Synch?

After the initial excitement over dating someone new wears off, you have to see if your daily lives are actually compatible. Strike a balance of coming together, yet still living your own life. At first, people feel so enthusiastic about the new relationship that they start to give up hobbies and habits in order to spend more time together. For instance, because my friend wants to constantly be around her new boyfriend who doesn't exercise, she hasn't been to the gym for six weeks. She's gained weight and is upset about it. Instead of sleeping late with him on weekends and going out for a big breakfast, she'd be better off sticking to her workout routine. In relationships you generally can't give up your healthy habits, hobbies, or passions for very long without becoming unfulfilled or resentful.

From the beginning, try to be the real you as far as what time you like to go to bed and what you like to eat and do for fun. Let's say a woman really enjoys her Wednesday evening yoga class, but that's one of the only weeknights that her new beau has free. She's tempted to skip it and go out with him. No, bad idea. People love people who pursue their passions, so pursue yours. Keep exploring your interests and being you. If he's a good match for you, he'll love to see you happy.

At this point in your relationship, you'll start to get a real picture of what your life together looks like. It's up to you to decide if you like what you see. Does he watch too much TV? Wake you up at 5:30 a.m. with a blaring alarm and then hit snooze every ten minutes? Leave dirty dishes in the sink? Behaviors can be worked on as everyone's comfort zones get pushed and budged, but certain tendencies probably won't change, so if it's a real struggle and you're constantly irritated by the way he approaches daily life, move on. Since real life only gets harder when kids enter the picture, jobs are lost, or a loved one dies, if real life with just the two of you is a headache, don't force it to work.

Time spent together versus apart can become an issue at this stage of dating. New couples often end up spending too much time together, which later makes it hard for people to establish their own boundaries. He wants to meet the guys for drinks, but you're like, well, what am I going to do? Friend time is very important, so let him have it. Meet up with friends of your own. Don't let excitement turn to clinginess, which then turns to suffocation. Always remember that you are an individual with a life beyond your relationship. Don't make the guy your whole world. Freedom is the best thing you can give a partner because it brings him back every time. On the flip side, you or he might be too busy with solo missions and may have to work on doing more as a team. The key is balance.

In a healthy relationship, it should be okay to make choices that aren't always what the other person wants to hear. He's hoping you'll join him for the Chargers game, but you already have plans. It's okay to say just that. You should be able to make an everyday choice without worrying about it turning into a fight or a big deal.

Drained or Charged?

Does this guy drain your energy? Bring you down? If you're more upset than you are happy—run, now. You also don't want a relationship in which you're always positive and trying to cheer him up. He's Mr. Down in the Dumps and you're Little Miss Pick Him Up, a one-woman band who's about to fall over from the strain. Relationships begin to fray when one person coasts while the other takes on most of the burden, whether it's emotional or physical. In healthy relationships, each individual charges the other. He makes you feel better after your rough day at the office, while you help him gather the courage to ask for a promotion. Like playing on a seesaw, a relationship's only engaging when both people put equal energy into it.

At times women feel like they aren't getting enough attention from a partner, which isn't a good sign. It shouldn't be a struggle for him to listen to and spend quality time with you. Unfortunately, women often act out in order to get the attention they're missing, which backfires. A common mistake is to play the sick card. A woman dramatizes how bad she feels and wants the guy to play nurse of the year. Honestly, go get some chicken soup, girl, and pull it together. Men don't want to think that their girlfriends have lousy health. Obviously you will occasionally get sick and he should be helpful, but don't exaggerate your condition or use it as a ploy to get attention.

Secondly, never be a drama queen. That is a horrible way to get attention, and men will find it irritating. Communicate what's bothering you and assert your needs and preferences. When he says he can't join you for lunch, don't flop on the couch crying and moaning and telling him he doesn't love you. (A) He's going to think you're a nutjob. (B) Men don't like feeling hopeless in the face of women's emotions. Express your emotions, but don't overplay them for manipulative effect. If you're truly not getting enough attention, he isn't a good fit for you. You should be recharging each other with love and communicating in a caring, honest manner.

When your boyfriend behaves in a way that you don't like, make sure you address it right away. A lot of women tell me their boyfriends or husbands are grumpy. Well, hello, ladies, it's because you've allowed them to be. If your boyfriend starts acting crabby, catch him off guard with a question like, "Wow, where did that come from?" He'll ask you what you're talking about. Say, "You're so negative today." He'll wonder, am I? "Yes, you really are. Life just seems like it's real tough for you today." Acknowledge the behavior in order to stop it, like you would with a kid with bad habits. Whether it's grumpiness, moodiness, a temper, or whatever, it's all about what the person is accustomed to and has gotten away with.

If you really care about him, bring attention to his behaviors that don't work for you. Men, like all of us, don't always see or realize what they're doing and what effect it's having. Or, they do and don't care to change. If that's the case, you need to ask yourself whether you can deal with their outbursts or whatever else they're doing that's bugging you. Probably not. It could be time to open that catalog again and start browsing for a better-tempered guy.

Meeting the Family

After about six months, if you haven't already done this, it's time to meet his family. I recommend a pre-meeting talk in which you get briefed on what to expect. He might tell you his sister is covered from head to toe in tattoos, his dad is hard of hearing and talks loudly enough to startle the cat, and his mom is a terrible cook so serve yourself small portions. Because I think it's a good sign when a guy truly loves and respects his mom, if he badmouths her in major ways (unless she really deserves it), be leery!

Meeting the family might reveal surprising truths about your new squeeze. His mom could tell you that your seemingly mild-mannered beau has really grown up since the time he was arrested as a senior in college for streaking drunkenly through the town square. Or that he was so scrawny and awkward as a teenager that he never had a girlfriend, and they worried he never would.

I know a guy named Doug who when meeting his girlfriend's parents for the first time found out from them that she owed them $50,000. Doug was taken aback to say the least. She explained that with job changes and unemployment she hadn't been able to keep up with the repayments. Doug later ponied up what she owed, and they got married, so even the things that catch you off-guard can work out in the end. The main point here is to pay attention to the startling statements that his relatives make, especially his parents! You can catch gems and juicy tidbits that will help you gain a larger perspective on your beau.

After you've actually met the family, be careful what you say. You can call your own daughter a brat, for instance, but you wouldn't like it if your new boyfriend did. The same applies to his family. Don't go on and on about the negatives. Were he to say, "My older brother is such a kook," it's better to laugh and respond, "He's pretty eccentric." Don't say, "Yeah, wow, who signed him out of the loony bin for today's reunion?"

Be sure to visualize yourself as part of the family. If they live in rural Arkansas, guess what? That's where you'll be going for the holidays. You have to decide if you like and respect his family and can see yourself interacting with them for years and years. If not, that might set off the warning bells. If you think to yourself, there's no way I am going to take a gamble on this DNA becoming part of my gene pool, then it's probably time to mosey on down the road or plan on adoption.

It's common that one person's parents are happily married, while the partner's family has a lot of problems. People from difficult backgrounds are often drawn to the stability of their partner's family. Your boyfriend might be trying hard not to live the way his dysfunctional family does, and you think that's a good thing. At other times, if your boyfriend's bad habits suddenly make a lot of sense when you meet his parents, you might decide that you don't want to stick around for the sequel.

Single parents: When you're ready to introduce your child to your new boyfriend, do it outside of the home. It's like putting a dog in another dog's territory; one is bound to feel threatened and act out. You don't want your child feeling uncomfortable in your home as he wonders if the guy is going to be around a lot or living there. So, incorporate your child into an interactive date, like miniature golf, on neutral ground. See how he gets along with your boyfriend. If they don't click well, it might take time or it just might not work out.

Unlike younger kids, teenagers are usually very slow to warm up to someone. They're already angry, defensive, and cautious. Don't try to force them to like your boyfriend. That won't work. They will respect people on their own terms and time schedule. If teenagers can tell that there is obviously a strong connection and that the guy is respectful and genuine, they will usually adjust. (I'll talk more about this in chapter twelve.)

If you want children, you need to ascertain whether your boyfriend also does by quietly observing his behavior around children. Does he play with your friends' kids or shoo them away when they get within five feet of him? Does he mention wanting children without you bringing up the subject? The worst thing that happened to my father was having us. He needed attention and once we popped into the world he couldn't get enough of it, so he looked elsewhere to find it. Loads of men will say they want kids, yet they don't behave in a way that actually supports that statement. As such, I suggest plopping your sister's baby on his lap and seeing what he does.

Don't Ignore the Red Flags!

In addition to testing out the guy's reaction to children and seeing if his family is a fit, you must pay attention to red flags. A red flag doesn't mean charge ahead like a bull—olé—it means danger, danger, run the other way! The situation that sets off warning bells in the beginning is often the one that ends the relationship. If he drinks too much now, he'll probably drink too much ten years from now. People can change, but you can't bank on it happening. Women will say, "He'll slow his drinking down once we have kids." Why assume that? You can try to influence other people's actions, but they'll only change if they want to. Point out what bothers you and then see if he takes proactive steps to improve it. If he doesn't, you have a decision to make.

I knew one of my husbands was bad with money. The first week we were dating he borrowed $200 from me. That should have gotten more of my attention. He also thought chivalry was hogwash. In the beginning of our relationship I waited for him to open my car door. He looked at me funny and asked, "What are you doing?" With all his physical aches and pains I think he was hoping I'd open the door for him. If that doesn't bother you, fine. That was a big red flag for me, though. And I just let that flag fly off the pole and drift away somewhere.

Looks are a bad vice. With the TDHs (tall-dark-handsomes), we get melted into the hair, the eyes, or the height and ignore the warning signs. I know I did. Not opening the door became not helping to carry the groceries that became me telling the hostess our name for the reservation while he stood indifferently off to the side. Borrowing money became chronic unemployment that became me being the breadwinner. Like many women, I thought things would change—that they'd get better. They didn't. Again, the red flags you see in the beginning of a relationship are often the behaviors that take it down, so don't rationalize your way around the telltale signs. Could I have done a better job reading the red flags? Yes, absolutely. That's a big reason why I'm writing this book. What I learned in hindsight through my various relationships can hopefully help you avoid similar mistakes.

Issues around money throw up more flags than a football referee. The guy might not be the contributor you thought he was going to be. You're dipping into your pockets way too much, and he's got alligator arms that never reach his wallet. Or he's self-consumed and has no problem buying himself a brand-new motorcycle, but you haven't seen a rose in a vase in a hundred years. Always keep in mind that money issues frequently ruin relationships. Irresponsible behavior and excessive drinking are other big red flags, but really a red flag is anything that catches your attention with a sinking feeling that says uh-oh. Don't ignore that feeling! Later you'll look back and say, "The signs were there all along. My gut was talking to me."

Keep in mind that everyone has a bad side. That bad side might never come out or very rarely emerge when someone is matched up well. On the other hand, a poor match can bring out the beast, and it is ugly to watch. A guy might be on an even keel in one relationship, for example, but another relationship with a more flirtatious, hardheaded partner brings out his temper. Pretty soon they're in weekly screaming matches and constantly pushing each other's buttons. If he's frequently flying off the handle, he's not the guy for you. Or if he brings out your bad side in a way that no one else has, he's not a good match. A temper (his and its effect on yours) is a big red flag to watch out for.

In your relationships, be clear about what you like and can stand. When you see a red flag, address it. Make sure it's a behavior he's willing to work on. If you don't deal with problems head on, the resentment builds, and you start to get mad about one thing after another. Once you start stacking all these issues, you blow or walk. He might not even see it coming. Men are so "left in the dark." I don't know a man in the world who needs a pair of sunglasses. When it comes to women, they are lights out all the time. A lot of that is because we don't tell them that our feelings are hurt, that we don't agree with their opinion, or that their behavior is unacceptable. You have to set a precedent for what you'll tolerate and won't, right away.

Women are afraid to speak up because they want so badly to be loved. They don't want conflict. To top it off, they are driven by a need to appear perfect to the guy. They think, "There's a thousand other girls out there. If I do this, this, and this, he's going to leave me." Believe me, ladies, from my matchmaking experience, I can tell you firsthand that guys will fight for the women they call feisty. They like a woman who has strong opinions. In fact, I've seen men purposefully try to get some fire out of their girlfriends who they think are too passive. Don't be afraid to voice your opinions and needs. He'll love you for it. And if he can't meet your basic needs, he's not good for you.

Normally you have to discover the red flags for yourself. Sometimes, though, men will test you, and the way that's handled can sound the warning bells. I recently talked to a 29-year-old woman who met a guy through the online dating service for Jewish singles called JDate. After dating and getting to know each other, the guy took her to The Gap and said, "I hope you know that if we got married, this would be the most expensive store where you could shop." He made a similar comment about a modest restaurant. I think he was just being practical and warning her—in a very unromantic way—about what he wanted in a marriage. This woman has lavish tastes that extend way beyond The Gap and Sizzler, but she was unwilling to walk away from him. Why? Because to her, he looked great on paper. Well, we aren't paper! We have personalities, and if she wants a higher-end lifestyle than what this guy says he's comfortable with, she should move on. It's up to you to the heed the signals, whether they're put out on purpose or accidentally!

Fighting Fair Versus Low Blows

Certainly by this point in the relationship, you're having disagreements. Those arguments can be good, as they allow you to define your boundaries. No one should be a doormat. But if those disagreements escalate into screaming, plate-hurling battles, duck—and then run out the door!

You have to stand up for your rights, but it's all in how you do it. As the saying goes, you get more bees with honey than vinegar. People need to work on being kinder to one another. I see in many relationships that couples spill a bunch of loud ugliness out of their mouths and then feel awful about it. Sometimes you'd rather have someone stick a knife in you than hear the things he said. Or if you're the one who did the verbal lashing, it's hard to wake up the next day and build a platform from that. You can say, "I love you and I didn't mean what I said." Well, there's a little bit of truth in everything we say, even if it's a joke, and you can't erase those words or take them back. They've been released and absorbed. If I hit below the belt with Robert, he would remember it forever. Some people have a file in their heads where they store everything negative that was ever said or done to them.

Many couples say to each other, "There's the door." That must be the biggest broken record. Once someone puts that out there, it's been set in motion. Both people are always going to be upset during a disagreement and considering storming out, or thinking the partner is going to storm out. If the guy is saying, "If you don't like it, leave," this threat tells you a lot about him; his perspective is black and white and he doesn't want to hear your side. When that's the case, you should walk through the door and close it behind you forever. Likewise, don't ever say that to anyone. My-way-or-the-highway is not a healthy approach. If you care about someone, you'll work on the issues in your relationship and vice versa.

Always keep in mind that words are dangerous, can devastate others, and can be used against you. So be careful what you say! Never call the other person a name. When in doubt, stick to talking about how you feel. It's not, "You're such a jerk! Why didn't you call me? I've been waiting for you for hours, you *&#$%!^!" Instead it's, "I felt really disrespected and hurt when you didn't call me to say that you couldn't make it. I was expecting you and waited three hours. Do you think that was a fair use of my time?"

If you're by yourselves, talk about the problem right away unless either or both of you are drunk, riled up, or very upset. Make sure you're both calm before trying to resolve the problem. If he's blowing up, let him blow. Remain quiet within yourself. Let that be over and don't say anything at that point. If you're the one who's all fired up, wait until the next day. Don't handle things when in a highly emotional state, because then it is likely the two of you will become louder and louder until the conflict builds into a screaming match. Some people, as soon as they're mad, want to get in your face right away, but it's horrible timing, because they're bound to say or do something regrettable.

When you're both calm, lovingly talk about what happened face-to-face. I don't believe in trying to settle conflict over the phone or through email. Get that person in front of you. Touching a person when you're talking to him is very important. If you can, hold his hand so he feels your physical warmth and love. Say, "I think it's really important that we talk about this. What can we do to make sure it doesn't happen again?" As he's talking, you can look in his face to gauge whether he's lying to you or being sincere.

It can be a major relief to release your emotions and speak your mind. Holding things in causes "dis-ease"/disease. Likewise, guessing what the other person is thinking is a waste of time. Stable people who are a good fit for each other can talk about everything and address conflict quickly rather than letting it stew. Truthfully, people can work through a lot when they care to. Many people just throw in the towel because they don't want to grapple with the issues that arise.

When you hurt his feelings, tell him you're sorry. If you aren't sorry for what you did, and this kind of situation happens repeatedly, then he's the wrong guy for you. In a good match, you shouldn't keep playing into the other person's hostilities. You both have to want to work on the things that trigger a negative response in the other person in order to make it through the inevitable obstacle course of life together.

Many women like to fight. It satisfies an urge in them, and then this usually backfires. If that's the case for you, when you start to get riled up, find a diversion. Go to the ladies room, play with your phone, or get some fresh air. Don't get into it with him. Wait until you are calm.

Experience has probably shown you that once you start winding yourself up, you blow and then antagonize the guy until he also blows. I've seen that a lot with friends. To appease certain women, men keep their balls in a drawer. But believe me, after enough provocation, those men are going to reach for those balls, and the result is not going to be pretty. All people have their breaking points; the key is not to trigger them.

There can be a lot of fighting when you're young, especially in your twenties, when partying can alter the dynamic and lead to trouble. At that age people aren't as ready to make major commitments and decisions, so they don't always treat their partner as well as they should. For couples of any age, fighting at times equals awesome make-up sex. Though that can be exciting, it can quickly become a bad yo-yo. You shouldn't need to fight to have great sex.

Watch out for other dysfunctional patterns that are easy to slip into, like the tit-for-tat habit. Because he did that, now I'm going to do this. You don't want to keep getting even, because it just perpetuates conflict.

Never get in an argument or criticize a guy in front of others! For men it's all about ego, the looking-good act. It could be the littlest thing, like telling him in front of his friends that his shirt does not go well with his pants. Men don't want to look stupid, incompetent, or be second-guessed, especially in front of others. Now, imagine a much worse offense than pointing out his mismatched clothes, when at a barbecue with his best buddies you start arguing about why he never pays for anything. Yikes! I can just imagine his wrath.

Men think, "If she has the guts to do this in front of my friends or family, then what's to come?" They imagine a snowball effect and see the disaster that will be their life looming on the horizon. Though that way of thinking might strike you as justified or melodramatic, the point is that guys want everyone to think they're wonderful, so if you screw up that image, they are ready to bolt. I ran into a couple recently who'd been married for over fifty years. I asked them what kept them together. They said it was the little things they've always tried to do for one another, respecting each other always, and never embarrassing each other in front of other people.

Despite the tough way they try to present themselves, men are delicate creatures. They are like roasted marshmallows—crusty on the outside, but warm and gooey on the inside. You have to realize that though it might not seem like it, your boyfriend is probably sensitive to criticism and conflict, so be careful about what you say and how you handle moments of frustration.

Also keep in mind that the less you try to control a guy, the more he'll love you. Why try to micromanage his every move? Likewise, the more controlling you get, the more conflict you'll have. You'll both start to feel drained, and the constant bickering will snuff out the flame of your love. Express yourself. Stick up for yourself. But don't attempt to manage all his comings and goings. If you don't trust him to make good decisions on his own, he's not the guy for you.

Get that plan in order, keep testing him, and handle conflict with such confidence and expertise that Dear Abby will fear for her job. Is he Mr. Right? Mr. Sort of Right? Mr. Yesterday's News? Let's jump ahead—with or without him—to the topic of engagement. If he's not the right guy for the aisle and the tux, you'll need to keep searching for the guy who is.

Let's look now at what's needed to take the leap of faith, as many people call it, though I prefer the term *trust your heart.*

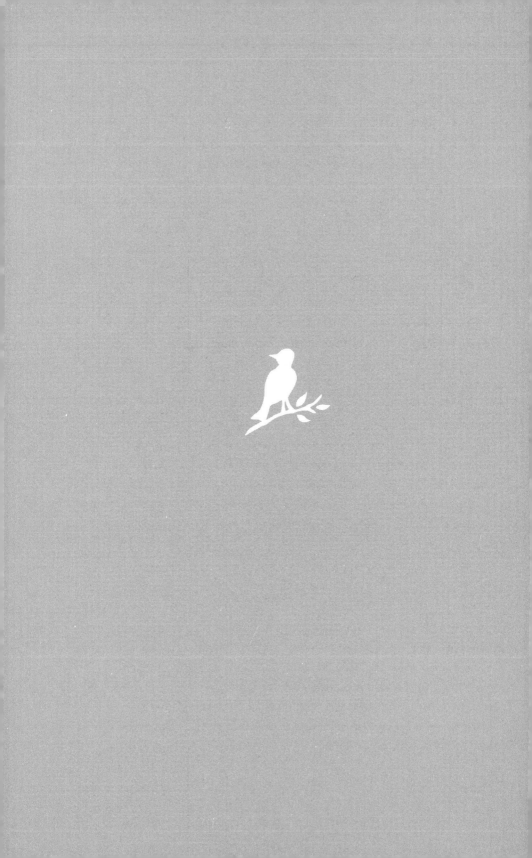

Trust Your Heart: the Marriage Leap

How do you decide if someone is right for you to marry? If he has a six-figure salary, muscular arms, and thick hair, does that mean he's golden? No, inevitably your heart gives you the answer. It's a feeling—an inspiration. Marrying him is a must. You can't picture yourself in the future without him, because he plays, and will continue to play, a major role in the movie that is your life story. He becomes you; you become him, and you "complete" each other like the famous line in *Jerry Maguire*.

People will ask: But how do you know there isn't a better fit? I think your heart, soul, and body tell you. You have the fluttering: he walks in the room and you get excited. You know that you can't let him exit your life; you have to seize the moment and make it happen. Imagining him with anyone but you is profoundly painful. You're not questioning who you are when you're in his arms. When he tells you he loves you, you know it—you don't suspect that he's lying or seeing someone else as soon as he leaves your side. It's a coherent trust and bond that both of you have, and it's magical. Love is magical.

To me, the whole objective in life is to collect as much love as possible before we leave this world. We have to trust what it is that we want and are striving for and just let our hearts give us the direction. If it's right,

113

then it's right. I don't care if you're twenty-five or seventy-five; people know when they're with a wonderful person and in a loving relationship. They feel cherished and want to keep the love fest going.

Engagement is that important last step before marriage that gives couples the chance to reevaluate whether "I do" makes sense. It's the time to solidify your love and the plans you've made together or to rub your eyes and say, "What was I thinking/drinking?" First, let's look at what it means to be married versus in a boyfriend-girlfriend relationship.

Why Get Married Anyway?

Let's say a friendly alien landed on Earth and wondered why some people wore gold bands and diamond rings on their left hands while others did not. If the curious creature journeyed around the United States closely observing people with and without rings, he would discover that a practice called marriage is an ongoing celebration of two people *who have a plan.*

Married folks tend to look into the future and give themselves direction. People living together are often going through the day-to-day motions without the shared mindset of: What are we going to be doing four years from now? Women know that if they ask their boyfriends that question, the subject of marriage will have to come up, and if that's not a topic that the guy wants to talk about, he's going to change the course of the conversation or get into an argument. Unlike some of your boyfriends, we'll return to this subject soon.

Marriage skeptics argue, "Why do I need a piece of paper or rings? I'm already committed in my heart. We have a strong bond." That can be true for a lot of couples, but it's often a copout for others. It may be considered very old-fashioned, but what is close to a woman's heart is a man taking the step of the "ultimate" commitment to marry her. The marriage proposal is never going to go out of style. And a girl who tells you, "I don't care if we ever get married," is, in my opinion, usually not telling the truth. There are exceptions of course. Some women who don't want children, for instance, might feel like marriage is unnecessary.

Marriage is a public declaration that two people want to share their moments (big and small), their lives, their children—everything— together as a couple. Why can't you achieve the same thing by living together? Because there's always the idea that it's not going to last. I mean, don't kid yourself: marriage can end. How would I know? Let me count the ways. But you have to jump through hoops to get into a marriage and even more to dissolve it, which generates a greater incentive to work on the relationship.

The same obstacles to breaking up don't exist in a boyfriend-girlfriend situation. No one has watched you stand in front of friends and family and say, "I do," so there isn't as much at stake. You might ask, isn't it better to stay unmarried, then, to avoid divorce? I think with stronger consequences come stronger rewards. The bonding and security that come with being married far outweigh, in my opinion, the possibility that it might not last.

When you have a boyfriend, you may not feel like he is really "yours." The revolving door is always there, and you're often wondering whether you or he will be walking through it. There's always some doubt. The uncertainty that stems from a lack of commitment can be very hard to deal with. Someone in the relationship usually wants more—at least eventually.

I personally never trusted men I dated until they started talking earnestly about marriage. Once that happened, I took them seriously and felt safe. The trust was there, as was the plan of moving forward together toward shared goals. Women don't trust men who don't mention marriage while in the boyfriend-girlfriend stage. The women think: I'm getting to know you for what reason?

I like marriage obviously. I love it! I think a marriage commitment is the ultimate in relationships. When I started dating after my first divorce, it was fun, but then as various relationships fizzled out after three months and most of the guys struck me as players who just wanted to have a good time and skate on, I felt empty. I wanted more.

Then Alex came along, who is nine years younger than I am, and we were crazy about each other. He didn't want children and was unconventional, so he suggested we have a "commitment ceremony" instead of a wedding. Since I was still reeling from my divorce and am pretty open-minded, I agreed to it, though I was lukewarm about the idea. Afterwards, people would ask, "What did we just witness? Are you guys married?" The confusion was awkward, and the commitment ceremony started to seem meaningless. As a result, a year later we formally got married in a courthouse.

Unfortunately for me, about one year after that, Alex changed his mind about children and wanted me to have a baby. My tubes were tied, and I had a daughter who was in her twenties. I thought long and hard about it, but just couldn't get myself to go through with it. Because I didn't want to prevent Alex from having the amazing life experience of raising children, we decided to part ways. It was an amicable, though heartbreaking, divorce.

Marriages can go in unforeseen directions. For instance, you would probably not expect that a partner would develop a gambling addiction or run off with your friend, but these things happen! Nonetheless, I think marriage is wonderful, and its benefits far outweigh the possibility of it not lasting forever. The love and bonding you feel, the everyday moments you experience with a person you love, the support you bring into each other's lives—everything from your husband getting you eye drops because your allergies are bothering you to helping each other deal with a loved one's death—all of that makes marriage a stable, caring foundation from which to approach life. If you've never experienced marriage, go for it. If you've been married before, do it again!

Balance Love and Practicality

Deciding to get married is not all about roses and love, however. There are many practical matters to consider before the proposal and while you're engaged.

It's time to get out your Dream Match List that I urged you to create in chapter three to see if you're staying true to it. You wrote it for a purpose! Sure, he might not meet *all* of its requirements, but don't just scrap the list because he's tall and has a sexy voice. On the other hand, if the guy has everything on the list but you don't love him, what kind of relationship is that? He could be perfect on paper (financially strong, wants children, has a good family, and so forth), but if you don't have the connection or fire and you can't cultivate it, you might as well take a flame and light up the list because it's not going to mean anything.

What if there's the fire without the list? Lord knows we've all been there. That happens more often than not. You want a little bit of both—fire and practicality. You can't have it all. It's a happy balance of making sure that the list holds true and that there's a strong romantic connection.

When people think about remarrying, they consider a lot of practical points, while young people taking their first plunge into marriage sometimes skip that step. The difference is experience. Someone who was married to a guy who was out of work for two years, drank too much, or did anything to bring about a lack of respect will not want to go down that road again, while a younger, never-married person won't have the same amount of hindsight to guide her.

These days, though, many people are waiting longer to get married and have children, which is often wise. It seems like the late twenties/ early thirties is becoming the new norm, as people hold off on marriage until they are fairly established. By contrast, in 1970 the median age for women marrying for the first time was 20.8. In earlier generations it was like, okay he's good-looking and terrific in bed, so let's tie the knot. Or, people married because the woman became pregnant and the proverbial shotgun got loaded. The oops/uh-oh situations can work out, but it's preferable to have a plan like the one we talked about last chapter.

Think again about the life plan you envision—no matter your age— and whether your guy can help you turn it into reality. His green eyes and captivating biceps aren't going to bring you financial security. Before getting married, you should discuss and agree on things such as who's going to pay for what, how many children you want to have, when you want to try for them, where you're going to live, and—if you're close to retirement age—what the plan is for the golden years.

Have you ever had a friend or family member who seemed out to lunch about the guy she was considering marrying? Women have a real knack for rationalizing and making excuses when they're in love. "Well, Harold is trying really hard to get a job. He just doesn't want one that starts early in the morning because he likes to sleep in. Harold said he will cut back on his drinking soon. I know he cheated on me, but he promised he wouldn't do it again." Meanwhile, you know that Harold is a lazy, lecherous drunk and you're wondering what kind of spell he put on your friend to keep her from seeing that.

Some people are in love with being in love and with the idea of marriage. They're equally afraid of being single and lonely. As a result, they may gloss over their partner's faults, make bad decisions, and rush into marriage without thinking things through. "I am not sure he's right for me, but he wants to marry me, so maybe I should marry him." Don't try to make the guy fit the marriage box; he should be a natural fit, not a contortionist.

The Marriage Practicality Checklist

Below is a quick, ten-point list of questions to ask yourself before getting married. For those of you who are engaged or are eyeing your partner as a future marriage contender, I suggest that after you read this section, you answer these questions on page 196 and jot down any hesitations or concerns.

1. Do you love him?

2. Do you think he'll continue to be a good fit for you in the future?

3. Do you have similar goals (regarding children, education, career, buying a home, etc.)?

4. Is he employed, financially stable, and responsible with money? Do you agree on who will pay for what, who will work, and how you will spend your money?

5. Do you have compatible views on childrearing, religion, and politics?

6. Do you communicate effectively with each other?

7. Are you comfortable around his family?

8. Do his everyday habits work for you?

9. Do you enjoy many of the same activities? Do you have similar active/inactive levels?

10. Does he have a life with friends, hobbies, and interests outside of yours?

These questions are pretty self-explanatory, and some have been covered in other chapters, so let's just delve in deeper on a few of them. Regarding #2, women have to look past the frivolous things (he sends me the cutest texts!) to what direction the guy is going to take. You need to think carefully about how happy and secure you'll be if you stay with him down the line. Maybe he's vacillated between college choices or dropped out and is enrolled in a culinary school. As a result he's racked up a lot of debt while flip-flopping between schools and never finishing anything. He's not sure he wants to become a chef now. You need to look at all that and not just fixate on the fact that he's a champion in bed and fun. You don't want a husband who can't see himself being a provider in any way or taking care of a child. Think about whether the guy has the potential to be a good fit in the future as your needs evolve.

Let the guy who's jumping from job to job and trying to find himself go through the process on his own. Then go back to him to see what he came up with. Don't be by his side with your binoculars trying to figure out what he's going to be when he grows up. I've been on that who-am-I safari with a couple of men, and it is exhausting. You become like his mom, maid, career counselor, and motivational speaker, and it just wears you down. Let the guy get the education, the job, and the plan before you make him the leading man in your movie.

Here's a note of caution if you want to have children: Certain men have personality types that can work one on one but not well as a family. I'm talking about the life-of-the-party, how-do-I-look-in-this-outfit? type. I call them peacock guys, and women flock to them. They're a blast and look fabulous on your arm. Trust me: I've had a few in my life. But they require a lot of energy. If you're willing to give them the praise and attention they need, they'll stay. My ex-husband Rick was a peacock, which is probably why I only raised one child with him. When you have a husband who needs a lot of attention or will otherwise feel neglected, forget about raising a big family together. If you're with a peacock, you're in his shadow as he does his dance and struts his stuff. You may not want to feel like the plain bird with beaks to feed who's wondering when he's going to quit flaunting his feathers! Remember, *there are the reason, season, and lifetime guys.* The key is knowing which category they fit into.

If a girl comes from a family that's done well financially—let's say her family owns a successful business—without always realizing it, she envisions someone continuing to support the lifestyle she grew up with. She expects her partner to be a financial provider who keeps the good times rolling. When she's dating the 6'4" guy who turns all the girls' heads, but his ambition is to be a painting contractor or a sales consultant at Pep Boys, she needs to think about the long-term effects of that job track. If it's really important to her that the guy be driven and make a lot of money, she should probably look elsewhere. Maybe she doesn't care about that or she wants to be the breadwinner, which could allow the relationship to work just fine. You have to know what you want and see how well it fits with what he brings to the table.

I hate to make marriage about money, but I would be a negligent matchmaker if I didn't warn you to pay attention to the almighty dollar. Money issues can tank a marriage! Before you get married, you need to discuss as a couple your financial plan. Who would work and at what capacity (full-time, part-time)? What is the savings plan? What are your assets, debts, accounts, and credit scores? Are you going to buy or rent? What is the monthly amount you could afford for a mortgage? If you want to be a stay-at-home mom, you need to make that clear and see if it's a possibility. If you're in law or dental school, he might expect that you'll always be working. Some women are corporate America and can't see themselves doing anything other than working, but maybe their husbands-to-be picture them staying home and raising the children. Don't let those desires be surprises! They can become major misunderstandings and frustrations down the line. Talk about finances ahead of time; make sure you're both in agreement and that the numbers add up.

Figure out who is going to handle all the bills and paperwork. If he is the one chosen to do this, you must make sure that you can check in at least once a month to review the statements and balances. I know a woman named Cynthia who thought she was in a financially stable marriage, but it turned out that her husband had a gambling problem and hadn't paid the mortgage in three years. Cynthia found out via a foreclosure notice on her front door.

These financial considerations are certainly not the stuff of romance novels. While feeding her grapes, the hunky protagonist doesn't start talking about his 401(k). But that's the difference between romantic fantasies and real life. In a marriage, you need the romantic and the real-life elements to fit together nicely. Without the practical parts in place, believe me, the passion will fizzle and your nerves will sizzle!

Following up on question #6 in the pre-marriage checklist, there's talking and there's communicating. A guy might talk to you about his day, but he doesn't listen when you talk about yours or seem to care what's going on with you. Words are bouncing around the room, but you're not really communicating. That's a very bad sign. In a marriage, you have to make a lot of decisions and adjustments, so you need to be sure that the two of you can express yourselves clearly and know you've been heard and respected. Along the lines of communication, ask yourself: Does he ever make you laugh? Laughter is really important! Be leery if he's too serious.

As for #10 in the checklist, don't enter into the commitment thinking that the other person is your whole world. As noted before, there's the famous line in *Jerry Maguire*: "You complete me." But, I would add: You're not my everything. You deepen what I already am. Men love independent, strong, decisive women who have a lot of friends. You shouldn't be his everything either. Encourage men to have friends and to do what they like to do, whether it's fishing, baseball, bowling, whatever. Whether you play it or he does, thank goodness for golf because it lasts for five hours and gives everyone a chance to get some space. I am all for women taking women time and men taking men time.

You might want to take a moment now if you're engaged (or hoping to be) to respond to the Marriage Practicality Checklist on page 196. Are you sure he's right for you?

Commitment Fears and Phobes

To say yes to a marriage proposal is all about trusting your heart and weighing in the practical considerations. Marriage is a statement that a couple can't live without each other and that both people are dedicated to making the relationship work. The rings signify the pledge to be faithful and to love each other without end.

Now, that commitment is not always easy to come by. At times tranquilizer guns and brainwashing sessions are needed. Why? Because men have a lot of fear! Guys are incredibly stuck in what they know. Anything outside of their box that they don't have firsthand knowledge of or know how to achieve frightens them. Men are also afraid of losing their freedom and getting burdened with responsibility.

Commitment-phobic men think that marriage equals boredom equals stagnant equals everything that's perfect going sideways, whether it's her attitude, looks, or productivity. They worry, for instance, that she's going to suddenly up and quit her job and have a baby, and then they're going to have to pay for it all forever and never get to do what they want. For them life is going to go to hell in her handbag. So for men reading this book who have the marriage jitters, rest assured that you can stay in a happy place. You have to learn to look at marriage as keeping the good times going. Focus on the now, and everything will fall into place if you stay true to each other and are committed to the relationship.

A young guy might not feel ready for marriage. He might want to sow his wild oats or collect enough dollars to create financial stability first. If he's committed to you but wants to wait, that's fine only as long as it's okay with you. But don't wait too long! Likewise, men who have been married before and have gone through messy divorces can be hesitant to try version 2.0, but again it's important to focus on your needs. I'm not a fan of women waiting for years for a guy to give them an answer. I have too much of an ego to sit around tapping my foot and staring at the clock, and I don't think anyone else should waste time either!

Of course, women can be the ones who hold out. They have second thoughts and see the red flags. And that's okay. The guy's not always Prince Charming. He might think she's the catch of a lifetime and that he needs to reel her in, but she might be saying to herself, "Uh oh, I don't know." Whatever the negatives are, women start hyperventilating. My friend Jodi was so frightened to tell her fiancé that she didn't want to get married that she had the moving crew come while he was at work and left him a long letter. Ouch! Women can be brutal. Please don't do what Jodi did! Be upfront and communicate directly.

There's also what I call the "white horse complex" that keeps people from heading down the aisle. It's common for young folks in particular to think that a white horse is going to pull up bearing a person who is better looking, wealthier, and more exciting. Though you don't want to settle for mediocrity, you also want to live in the present and seize the opportunity in front of you before it's gone.

For some long-time bachelors, the right girl changes everything. But some of them just never will make a marriage commitment, and you're better off without them. Most men and women want to get married, however. I think that the really responsible guys, once they're connected with a great match, can discuss marriage openly and execute their masculinity by popping the question without needing to be nudged. They can say things like, "I knew I wanted her to be the mother of my children, and I had to act." But I'd say about seventy-five percent of guys need at least a little sweet-talking. They have to be spun around and given a little push in the right direction. Men are in a rush professionally, but they're not usually hurrying to start a family. Women, on the other hand, feel the pounding of their biological clock and may want to nest and feel secure.

Remember the one-and-a-half-year rule from last chapter? You should be engaged within a year and a half of dating. If that time passes with no engagement, have a heart-to-heart talk with your boyfriend. Either he has no intention of getting married or the love's not that strong. Don't hang yourself out to dry. Some women are too wimpy about getting commitments. If the heart-to-heart talk doesn't create movement, then lace up those walking shoes and hit the pavement. If he really wants to marry you, he'll come after you.

I know a woman named Tania who stayed with a guy for seven years and kept trying to get him to go down the aisle. He'd dangle carrots, but he never popped the question. Fed up from being strung along and unwed, Tania, thankfully, finally left him. She was heartbroken, but she didn't want to waste any more time waiting for a commitment that time proved was never going to happen. Don't let that be you!

What can you do to avoid Tania's situation? Remember, ideally you're dealing with a one-and-a-half-year window, so don't kick the can down the road for years and years. Instead, within the first six to nine months of dating, test your boyfriend. When his guard is down, like after sex, ask him hypothetical questions such as: If we got married, where would you want to live? Since you grew up with a big family of four siblings, would you also want to have a large family? The way he answers or sidesteps these types of questions tells you a lot. It's a bad sign if he immediately tries to change the subject or says, "I don't want to talk about this." If asking these questions causes an argument, that's also a red flag. Commitment-phobic men are masters of avoidance and deflection.

Often women don't say anything because they're afraid to rock the boat. They think if they mention the word marriage or start to pressure him, the guy is going to run or get defensive or think of a hundred excuses why they shouldn't be having this discussion. But just because she's not asking doesn't mean the guy's skating. That's a very bad misconception. Men don't always realize that the woman cares about getting married because she never expresses that desire to him.

But let's say you have talked to your boyfriend about your desire to get married and he has turned into the proverbial deer in the headlights who's making you hit the brakes and skid off the road. First of all, there's a difference between nudging and forcing. You don't want to wear the guy down like a torture victim until he finally says, "All right already, I'll marry you!" That's the last thing you want. The skittish guy who has to be pushed into marriage will have to be pushed into everything. You need to make sure he's genuinely excited even if initially it takes him time to overcome his fear.

Men, like all animals, can be trained. Paint a bright, enthusiastic picture of your lives together and your boyfriend will start to admire the view. Women have to be salespeople. Make your shared future a vision that warms his heart. "Honey, if we got married we could take that two-month trip to Europe that we've been talking about and buy that house we've been eyeing on Lover's Lane." Nagging, on the other hand, will backfire. A rosy dream of you enjoying life together will get him to melt like a popsicle. If it doesn't, he might not be a good match or marriage material. Next!

Live Together Once You're Engaged

In general, if marriage is your goal, I don't believe you should live with a partner unless you're engaged. I say this for two reasons: (1) The guy thinks: Why buy the cow when you can get the milk for free? (2) It takes away the excitement of living together once you're engaged and married. A man is often unmotivated to propose if you're already living together, because he has a perfect situation: 24/7 access to you without all the responsibility of marriage.

That being said, I don't want to make living together a black-and-white scenario because it's not. I know many couples who lived together first and then got married, and it worked out well. I've seen other couples who never got engaged because they found too much fault with each other while living together, which means it was a good test for them.

My best advice is to sandwich the living-together stage between two commitments. You start with getting engaged, the first commitment, which leads to moving in together and planning a wedding. I recommend that you find neutral ground: a new house or rental together. If you own your own homes, keep them. Turn them into rentals until you see how it all pans out. Then once you've lived together, you can get married, the second commitment. That way everything is in forward motion.

But I definitely don't advise not living together before marriage. I've seen that really backfire. Jennifer, a woman with strong religious principles, lived in her own place until the wedding, but six months after the wedding the relationship went sideways. Why? Because she and her husband didn't really know each other's habits or how to interact with each other on a daily basis. It was all a fantasy and they couldn't do real life together because they never actually experienced it. Dry running a situation is a good thing to do. Practice makes perfect, whether it's sex, living together, or throwing darts.

During that trial engagement period of cohabitating, make sure the guy is capable of doing real life. If he's still living like a bachelor, and nothing's changed except that you sleep under the same roof, that should give you pause. You're not going to make him give up his band or nights out with the guys, but you should sense that he's making time and opening up his life for you and vice versa. At this stage, bad habits that had gone unnoticed can start to cause concern. You didn't know he smoked pot so often, for instance, or that he gets irritable easily and has mood swings. Pay attention to all of these behaviors. Have his family over and invite your family over. See how these various scenarios play out because it will give you insight into what marriage with him will be like.

A lack of communication is one of the biggest reasons why couples don't make it when they move in together. Along those lines, you can judge how well it's going by how often you're fighting. You could be fighting about little things, like no one is going grocery shopping or he invited a bunch of guys over without telling you, and you didn't discover the sausage fest in your living room until you walked into the hallway in your bathrobe. Those little things turn into big things quickly. Money easily becomes an issue too. You may have thought he was going to pay for everything; he thought you were going to cover half. Or you start resenting that you're buying all the food and covering the utility bills, and this was not part of the agreement. Real life presents itself, which causes problems. You have to talk through those issues to determine whether better communication and a few behavior changes or adjusting expectations can solve the problems, or if you're just not compatible enough to get married.

Let's say things appear to be going well, but the wedding is still nowhere in sight. Beware of the engagement trap. Several years can go by with no wedding and the woman's wondering, "Are we ever going to get married? Did he just put the ring on my finger so that I'd move in with him?" Some guys do that. He buys the ring to shut her up; she won't be bitching at him about getting married, and her parents see the engagement as justification to live together. I don't like any of that. It's a big game to some men until the woman blows the whistle. I know a couple in that situation right now. I ran into them in a restaurant parking lot recently, and when I noticed the big rock on Wendy's finger, I gave them a hearty congratulations and asked when their wedding would be. Don, who is quite the manipulator, said, "All right, Barbara, that's enough. One step at a time." They'll probably never get married. Don will keep coming up with excuses why it's not the right time, but later will be. I just hope Wendy figures that out and blows the whistle.

Remember the plan! Within a year of getting engaged, have the wedding. Don't let yourself get strung along.

The Vows

I, (name), take (name), to be my lawfully wedded (husband/wife), to have and to hold from this day forward, for better or for worse, for richer or for poorer, in sickness and in health, to love and to cherish, till death do us part.

Personally, I think the original vows that were laid down many years ago should be tweaked, because "till death do us part" is a big command that strikes me as a little nuts. Ideally we'd like to be with someone forever, but it doesn't always work out that way. I don't think we should punish or fault ourselves if we can't live up to the vow of lifelong matrimony. In my opinion, "till death do us part" should be changed to "till a lack of life do us part." I don't think people should stay in relationships where the love and respect is gone, where misery is a constant companion, where cheating is rampant, and so forth. I don't think it's wise to take the mentality that come hell or high water, you will never get divorced. I think you have to evaluate a relationship on a daily basis to see if it's actually good for you. You work to change the things you can; you adapt and communicate, but please don't ever settle for misery. It's just not worth it. When marriage becomes the death sentence to your happiness, how holy and sacred is it? Say vows that are true to your heart and that you both want to live by, whether they are the traditional ones or not.

The main focus is to make what you believe are good choices and not ever feel like you're stuck. Be present, be fresh, be exciting. Care, communicate, and grow together. Enter into marriage with the intention of loving someone forever and give it your best shot for as long as possible. Maybe that'll be a lifetime. As we'll discuss next chapter, a good marriage gets better when you continually put energy into making it exciting rather than slumping off into the doldrums.

Stoke the Fire: How to Keep the Spark in Marriage

THERE'S THE FANTASY WEDDING, the romantic honeymoon, and the exciting first year of marriage. Beyond that timeframe, it's often accepted that marriage becomes boring and marks the end of your fun social life. Wrong! Why would you want to live that way? In this chapter, we will look at ways to keep your marriage exhilarating throughout the years.

Anything or anyone you love requires time and energy, which means you have to work to keep a relationship thriving. When you put effort into something—whether it's your brain, body, artwork, or marriage—it will get better. That's the first rule for keeping the spark in marriage: be ready to put energy into your relationship. Otherwise, it will certainly get stale.

Marriage skeptics will say, "Marriage is an institution," or "marriage is boring." Guess what? If you think that way, you will feel that way. You create your own mindset and lifestyle.

It is up to you to insert the fun back into marriage and keep the momentum going to ensure that life feels fresh and interesting. I realize that paying bills is not fun; nor is having a premature baby. There are definitely stresses that will arise in marriage, but when the respect remains strong between you and your husband, and you are both dedicated to weathering the inevitable storms, you will find marriage to be a great comfort. Together you are better! And when the sun starts to shine again, take advantage of the opportunity to show each other how important your love is.

Keeping the spark in marriage is about surprises of all kinds. It's about newness and motion and energy. It's about planning and communicating with care and respect. It's about separating the "tender" from the "trap" because you are never stuck in marriage. Marriage is a choice that, when approached with a positive outlook, can be rewarding beyond your wildest dreams!

Let the Excitement Continue Beyond the Aisle

My daughter had a huge, elaborate wedding with her first husband. On their honeymoon, he asked, "So now what?" Too often that is the deflated way that people transition from a wedding into marriage. A marriage party is never over. We should always strive to be festive in our relationships.

With a $70-billion-dollar business sector fueling the march down the aisle—from florists to reception halls to deejays and so forth—the planning and presentation of a wedding can be a blast, especially for women. You've got the dress, the veil, the invitations, the champagne, the twinkle lights. Yay! Though there can be many stresses and headaches along the way, planning for the wedding is an exciting process that puts your engaged life in blissful forward motion.

Then, after you stand up in front of family, friends, and colleagues to declare your love and intention to forge a life together, you hopefully go on an amazing honeymoon. When you return, you have a new home to decorate as presents arrive from the wedding registry. Soon after, you start trying for a baby. Typically, then, the first one to three years of being engaged then married go really fast. It's always about what's next. Next! And that keeps your married life in motion.

Everything goes pretty well in marriage when there's something to look forward to. But then, let's say your children are five and seven years old, and you're not planning to have a third. You may start wondering,

Now what? I'm bored. Is this it? Nobody likes feeling stuck in the doldrums questioning where her life is headed. It's up to both people in a marriage to keep things moving. Whether it's planning for children, trips, family reunions, dates with your husband, or volunteer activities, the whole idea is to give yourselves reasons to be invigorated. You want your life to play out as a movie in your mind and see greatness always in the making, building scene by scene.

Let's play the "m" game. I want you to associate *marriage* with *movement, motion,* and *momentum.* One of the basic laws of physics is the law of inertia: "A body at rest remains at rest . . . unless acted upon by an external force." If you don't put any energy into your marriage, it will stay the same. It's not going to stir on its own. You need to get it up on its feet and in motion. Let's take a look at how to make that happen.

Give yourselves something to look forward to.

Get events on the calendar—large and small. From planning for babies to a romantic weekend in the mountains to a girls' dinner out, both of you need to mark the calendar with events that make you smile just thinking of them.

Plan, and do!

If you don't plan, you don't do. Since it takes time and effort to make dinner reservations, buy tickets to a play, look up directions, and get dressed up, people don't bother. But believe me, if you're feeling stuck in a boring relationship, you need to step up your game and start scheduling social events. It doesn't matter what your budget is, you can find plenty of free or expensive things to do: street fairs, hikes, brewery tours, or five-star dinners. It's all about tailoring things to your taste and budget and cultivating a zest for life.

The "what are we doing this weekend?" question gets old, and women often feel disappointed when one predictable weekend leads to another and then another. On the other hand, I've found that men rarely want to do the last-minute plans that women come up with. Robert, for instance, doesn't do "spontaneous" well. It's not part of his personality. When men begrudgingly follow women's last-minute plans, there's friction created that can last the whole weekend. So, do yourself and your marriage a favor and make plans ahead of time!

Put the time in.

No one is too busy for romance, and all couples need to devote time to celebrate their love. Enjoy a concert in the park together. Pick up a sweet card, write a nice note inside, and leave it on the front seat of your husband's car so that he sees it on his way to work. Surprise him with a bottle of wine, an appetizer spread, and lively music when he walks in the door after a long day. Or drape a bathrobe on the bed and have aromatic bath salts ready for a relaxing soak.

Anything that shows that you have taken the time to think of your husband's needs goes a long way. Let's say he mentions in an off-hand way that he needs workout socks. Think how pleased he'll be a day later when you present him with a new pack of socks without his asking. When you show your husband love and affection, he will likely do the same. You can also be more forward. When there is seductive energy between you and your husband, playfully tell him that you're looking for something super romantic to happen in the next forty-eight hours.

Mix it up.

Marriage can equal "old." Not old in age, but blah. People often let their marriages get too routine, too predicable, too freaking boring. Every weeknight when the kids go to sleep, the couple watches television and drinks a glass a wine. That's great part of the time, but every Monday through Friday night? Yikes!

Structure and routine are good to a certain extent, but don't let them become suffocating. You build structure for the health of your family. Young children especially need a lot of structure such as set bedtimes and mealtime routines. But don't let that structure carry over into *all* aspects of your life—you're not four years old—because it will cause monotony in your marriage.

Instead of watching television yet again, have friends over to play poker. Or take a moonlit walk. Give each other massages. Take an hour or two to feed your creativity, whether it's painting, writing, wood carving, playing guitar, or whatever. Mixing things up is like shock therapy for your relationship.

Breaking up the routine even in tiny ways can add joy to your lives. Eat dinner in a different part of the house than you're used to. Leave the bed unmade on Sunday so that you can easily find your way back into it. Light a scented candle next time you watch a movie at home together.

The world of two people can become way too small in a marriage. Let's say you've got your country club, the two restaurants where you always go, and the park where you walk the dog. With many activities to choose from wherever you live, broaden your world and try new spots. Take a day trip or a cooking class together. Get creative.

Change things up for yourself, too. One day a week, do things a little differently. Eat foods you don't normally eat; drive a different way to work; watch a documentary you normally wouldn't choose. Getting outside of the box in your individual life helps you to break out of the box as a couple. If you dress conservatively, get a wilder outfit. If you dress provocatively, tone it down for a change. Don't be overly predictable.

Keep the dating in marriage.

All of the creativity and romance that go into dating are often thrown out the window during marriage. *Marriage should be permanent dating with the same partner*, and it should be the best of the best! Plan fun, romantic outings with each other on an ongoing basis.

Robert and I have date-night once a week. It is my responsibility to plan an outing one week, and the next week it is his. Try it in your relationship, and every once in a while attempt to create anticipation before your date like, "I'm taking you somewhere special at noon. Be ready with comfortable walking shoes and bring a bathing suit." Not knowing what's coming next gives people a thrill.

Bring on the romance.

My friend Linda told me about her brother Fred who, after over thirty years of marriage, is still as romantic as ever. For Valentine's Day, he presented his wife with gifts at various moments throughout her day. At first they were small things, like a new lipstick. Then in the evening, Fred gave her an elegant dress to wear at dinner. When they returned home from the restaurant, he asked her to wait in the car. He went inside and lit candles and scattered rose petals along the staircase and into the bedroom. Fred led her up the candlelit walk and had a final gift waiting for her: a sexy negligee.

Now, as Linda explains, Fred and his wife have had their problems. It hasn't been all roses and candlelight, but their loving gestures to each other are an investment in their family. Linda said to me, "Sometimes I wonder if I had done things like that in my marriage if I'd still be married to my first husband." Who knows the answer to that question? In some cases no amount of romance can save a relationship, but other times it can provide the spark needed to reignite the passion that's been there all along.

Get out of ruts.

When you lose laughter and romance and playfulness, a marriage can fall apart. As we'll talk about in future chapters, there are times when the problems in your relationship are too big to overcome. But what I am talking about here is getting out of the ruts that are easy to fall into. You haven't walked on the beach together in twenty years and you miss those days. Well, it's not too late. Men (and women) can be trained to have better habits. It's all in your approach.

Not walking on the beach has become the norm for your husband, but it doesn't have to stay that way. I would start off by saying to him in a friendly way, "I was just thinking the other day of how we used to take long sunset walks on the beach at Torrey Pines. Remember the time when . . . ?" As your conversation continues, offer with enthusiasm, "Why don't we go for a walk on the beach this Sunday? That would be wonderful!" If your husband has a lot of love and respect for you, he will make an effort to make you happy. If he doesn't automatically agree to the walk, tell him that on a future date it would really please you. Let it go, and I'll bet that he follows up later.

Keep in mind that to a certain extent you have to accept the individuality of the person you're married to and vice versa. If he's painfully shy, you're probably not going to convince him to celebrate Mardi Gras on the streets of New Orleans no matter how much he wants to please you. Try to understand what your husband will and won't do and be reasonable. But, never be a doormat, and don't settle for mediocrity! Unless your husband has serious physical limitations, taking a walk on the beach is completely doable.

People don't respond well to being criticized, so you **don't** want to say, "You used to be such a romantic guy. What's happened to you?" I'll explain why later in the chapter, but your approach with men is of the utmost importance. Also keep in mind that men will assume that you are fine with the way things are if you haven't said anything to indicate that you're not. Guys get quite comfortable in their routines, which often involve a clicker, a sport, or a cocktail (or a combination thereof) and they lose perspective on how interesting or uninteresting your daily life is together. The view from the man cave is dim, so throw him a bone and tell him there will be more where that came from if he joins you for a romantic walk.

Make the little things count.

You don't need to have elaborate plans all the time to feel content in your marriage. Sometimes it's just nice to know that your husband is picking up the kids from school and paying the electric bill. It feels good to count on someone. His responsibility puts you in a happy place and vice versa. The little things you do for each other go a long way—making coffee in the morning, for example, or dropping off the dry cleaning. Being with a responsible and thoughtful partner is a godsend that saves you from a lot of stress.

I've had female clients whose ex-husbands owned Maseratis and Ferraris and took them on lavish vacations once a year, but the rest of the time their husbands were jerks. Those luxury vacations and vehicles—big-ticket items—don't make up for the bad behavior and lack of respect for all the other weeks of the year. It's the every-day respect, positive attitude, and caring outlook that matter. The little things that show that two people care about and are dedicated to each other go a long way.

Steer clear of the comfort trap.

I hate the expression "letting myself go." Too often people stop taking care of themselves when they're married. They become inactive and gain lots of weight. At that point, they're not "letting" anything go; they're keeping everything from going. People often say to me, "We just got comfortable with each other." Well, get uncomfortable. If that's what comfortable looks like, I don't want to wear it, whether it's ugly sweatpants or twenty pounds of extra weight. Sitting around eating bonbons, not exercising, never going anywhere, and watching TV every night will not make you happy. There has to be some kind of stimuli that keeps people excited about being with each other. No one wants a blobby existence.

And don't kid yourself: men care what women look like in the same way that women care what men look like. My friend's sister was upset because her husband wanted her to lose weight. She said, "What does it say about a man if he only accepts you when you look a certain way?" My friend replied, "It says he's typical." Love runs deeper than appearance, but when someone's good looks fade due to laziness, it does not help to keep the spark alive. It's never too late to get moving, to practice portion control, to start an exercise routine, or update your wardrobe—whatever it is that you need to do to get your shine again. Start small and be consistent; over time you'll see big changes.

Get your sexy back.

I don't care if you have more skills in the kitchen than Martha Stewart—in order to draw and keep a guy's interest, you need sex appeal. Women must feel that power and project it. It doesn't matter if you've slept with two people your entire life or two people in a single day, sex appeal is all about the power of suggestion. No matter how long you've been married, your husband will love it when you get your sexy on.

Men like to chase things. They like to chase footballs, promotions, and women. So give your husband the sensation that he's chasing you, whether it's around the bed, up the stairs, or in his mind. Get flirty and suggestive and just tantalizingly out of reach.

Bring on the romantic foods such as chocolate, strawberries, oysters, and champagne. Ask your husband to tell you or write down three things that turn him on, and you do the same. It can be something small like a kiss on the nape of the neck to something kinkier—whatever works for you. Buy new lingerie or other forms of inspiration.

I also suggest that couples make and exchange love coupon books. For example, a coupon could be good for a nude swim in the pool, a bubble bath for two at 8 p.m. with champagne, his favorite lasagna dinner, or his favorite sexual position. With the coupon books, ask for whatever it is that you yearn for in the privacy of your mind and inspire him to do the same.

Be free to be you and to have your own space.

I once met a yoga instructor named Chelsea who shared with me her belief that marriage gives you the freedom to be yourself. She said marriage is like being in a yoga position in which you're grounded at your base, which then frees your upper body to really stretch and move. I loved her analogy!

Knowing that someone loves and emotionally supports you gives you tremendous freedom to express your own individuality. So take time to be you. Explore your passions. No one is meant to be with another person twenty-four hours a day, seven days a week. But what happens in marriages is people get clingy. Don't be smothering. Let your husband have time to hunt or kayak or read, and enjoy the same freedom for yourself. Let him have his guys' weekend; you go on a girls' weekend. Space and time away are very healthy for both of you and give you perspective on why you love the other person. The foundation of a good marriage is celebrating each other for who you are apart and together.

Loving Communication, Not Verbal Combat

One surefire way to douse the flames of love is to get into ugly, insult-hurling arguments. Heated fights can lead to fiery sex, but they don't usually make you feel great about yourself. With two people flying off the handle and blaming each other for the problems in their marriage, hurtful things get said that are hard to forget. As I discussed in chapter nine, it's important to stand your ground but in a respectful way. After all, the idea is to be heard and understood, not resented and avoided. Caring communication is vital to keeping the spark alive in your marriage.

Marriage is two people contributing all the time. The respect has to be there in order for the relationship to work. If it's not, you're just putting Band-Aids on a cut that's bleeding when you need stitches. In many marriages, respect is the answer to how long the relationship will last. When admiration and courtesy are present, you can handle things that come up and also avoid each other's triggers.

Before you say a word to your husband about what's bothering you, ask yourself if what you're about to say is respectful. Would you want to be spoken to that way? If there's any doubt, rephrase it. Satisfaction in a marriage stems, in large part, from love and respect.

It's never too late to change your approach, reaction, or behavior. So if you've been an irritating nag lately and you've noticed that your husband stays as far away from you as possible, switch it up. Try complimenting him or doing something nice. He might be shell-shocked at first or think it's a trap, but eventually he'll come within ten feet of you especially if you dangle food scraps. But in all seriousness, when there is still respect in a marriage, you can choose to go to what I call your happy place—a state of mind in which you feel gratitude and love toward your husband. When you go to your happy place, you help him to do the same.

Help your husband to shine rather than pointing out the tarnish.
Marriage falters when two people put each other down, and it flourishes when two people empower each other. Men respond very well to attention and very poorly to accusations and insults.

I have found that women like to resent men; it gives us a good reason to be a bitch. The problem is that this power trip backfires because the blame game doesn't work. He's *never* going to stand there and sincerely say after you've yelled at him, "You're right. I am a lousy husband who is lazy, inattentive, insensitive, and dull." What will happen is that he'll get defensive, angry, and insulted. He'll blow up at you in greater fury and avoid you for days. How is that good for your relationship?

Sullen, unspoken blame doesn't work either. My friend was complaining to me recently about her lousy sex life with her husband. She completely put the blame on him and his performance, but she hadn't attempted to communicate her wants to him or to take proactive steps to improve the situation. I suggested that she work with him, be supportive, and try to create some fire. I don't care if a couple hasn't had sex in ten years, they can take action to get things moving again—literally!

What you need to keep in mind is that in these kinds of scenarios, it's not just his problem, it's hers, too. We all get stuck and need new energy. We have to take gentle care of each other's egos and inspire each other. In the same way that you don't want anyone to make you feel bad about yourself, he doesn't want to be made to feel bad about himself.

Always keep in mind that in a relationship *it takes two*. If you think your marriage is boring, you are just as responsible for that as your husband. It's up to you to make things happen, just as much as it's up to him. Instead of fixating on what he is or isn't doing, see what role you can play to improve the situation.

Pull your weight, and inspire your husband to do the same. Assign him certain responsibilities if you feel like he's not doing enough. "It would really help me out if you could take Nate to school on Wednesday mornings. That way, I can get Kiera to daycare on time. Do you think you could do that?"

Also, don't make your husband feel bad about his attempts to impress or help you. If he changes the baby's clothes and put the pants on backwards, don't berate him or he'll never perform that task again. Thank him for helping and if it's really important to you, show him in a nice way how those pants go on. At times, though, it's better to be silent than right. Think about it: Is anyone actually going to notice that your four-month-old has her pants on backwards? Is she going to feel the difference? No, so it might not be worth pointing it out to him. Since men hate feeling inadequate, when you want their help don't be a supreme critic. I know it can be annoying dancing around their delicate egos, but it's much better than the alternative of upsetting their sense of self-worth.

Compliments of any kind are really important for the health of a relationship. We want to hear that we look good in our new clothes, and our husbands want to hear that the dinner they cooked was delicious. Compliments make people feel noticed and cherished. When you feel negative or stagnant energy setting in, offer up a sincere compliment.

If men had tails, it would be easier to know their dispositions. Oh, look, it's wagging! He must have gotten that new client! Though it's not always clear what your husband is thinking, you can get to know him very well, which helps you to avoid needless drama. Think about what works with him and what doesn't in order to anticipate how best to approach him. Give your husband the opportunity to shine rather than thrusting a task on him that will not go over well because of the situation or timing.

For example, if you know that he is usually exhausted when he first comes home from work, don't make that the time to ask him to move the couch. Maybe mentioning it to him before he goes to bed and suggesting a time to rearrange the furniture in the next day or two is a better approach.

Lastly, let his balls be there. If you override your husband and constantly nitpick him (there's a big difference between standing up for yourself and being a pain), he's going to feel emasculated. You don't like being told what to do all the time either. So pick your battles and let him play with his balls.

Be positive in your own mind.

As I've said before, your subconscious mind can't take a joke and accepts what you say as reality. When you tell yourself that your marriage is boring, you hear it, believe it, and perpetuate it. You become what you say. When you start to complain about the job you hate, the house that's too small, and the children who don't mind you, you get yourself more and more stuck in a negative cycle.

Use the power of the mind to create beneficial changes. If you're feeling like your life is crappy, say, "I am no longer going to live this way. Tomorrow I will start looking for a better job and putting a discipline plan in place for the kids." Loving communication is not just between you and your husband; it is also the messages you send internally about your marriage, so be careful and conscious about what you say—whether it's aloud or in your mind.

Let your enthusiasm do the talking.

If I have enthusiasm for an idea, Robert will usually go along with it even if he initially considers it unappealing. For instance, the year that my father died, Robert asked me where I wanted to go for New Year's. I hoped to visit St. Louis, the area where my father lived and I grew up, and have that authentic Midwest Christmas experience with the snow and the cold. When asked, I presented the idea to Robert with a lot of gusto, and although I knew he wasn't going to be thrilled—he's from New York and prefers to leave those cold winters behind—the next day he said, "We're all set. I bought the flights, and we're going." I got to connect with my hometown and the memory of my father, and I was very grateful to Robert for understanding and making it happen.

Start with enthusiasm and you'll be amazed where it takes you. Guys want to please their gals, and your excitement is their obvious cue that what you're requesting truly matters to you.

Don't nag.

Just say what you want in a friendly, upbeat way. "Honey, let's see a play! Wouldn't that be fun?" would get a better reaction from your husband than a whiny-voiced, "We haven't been to a play in ages. We never do anything cultured anymore."

To nag is to "annoy or irritate (a person) with persistent fault-finding or continuous urging." When you nag, your husband feels drained before he's even started, and you feel irritated. We're not always in the mood to say things in a nice way, but it requires more energy to apologize and clear the air if you get too snappish. Also, when you're constantly nagging, you send the signal that you want out of the relationship because you keep finding many faults with your husband. Is that the signal you want to send? If not, pay attention to your triggers and hold back the urge to yell at him to take out the damn trash already! If you haven't noticed, nagging doesn't work well with men anyway. They just tune you out or defy you, and they are very good at that.

Don't go to bed mad.

Clear the air before you go to bed. Never go to bed mad because you will wake up mad and eat your breakfast mad. You end up building a fortress around you that leaves you isolated and upset. My advice is to always nip the issue in the bud. Communicate how you're feeling and try to fix the situation. If he's stubborn and caused the problem in your opinion, I suggest taking one for the team. Say, "I am upset about the way this evening has gone, and I'm sorry we didn't handle this situation better. What can we do to get back on track?"

Some readers might be thinking, Barbara, you're stuck in the sexist past. Why do I have to take the fall or do all these things for my husband? What's he doing for me? I understand that way of thinking, but here are my thoughts on the matter: One of you has to back down. If you're worried that it will always be you, take heart. In my opinion, your husband will notice that you're always compromising, and he will start to pick up the slack and do the same. You'll influence his reaction to a fight by being a good example. If he doesn't eventually put in the effort or show you respect, then he should be replaced by someone who will.

Keep good influences around you.

Misery loves company. If you want to be in a good relationship, hang out with others who are in a good relationship. If you hang around with couples where the guy talks down to his wife or she talks down to him, next thing you know you start absorbing their bad behavior. We learn from the people we spend time with. Just think how much more you tend to complain about life when you're with that friend who is always griping. Your spirit will sink or rise to the level around you.

Next up: they whine, they cry, they try your patience, but they are ultimately incredibly rewarding. Am I talking about men? No, but that's a good guess. I am referring to humans even more helpless: children.

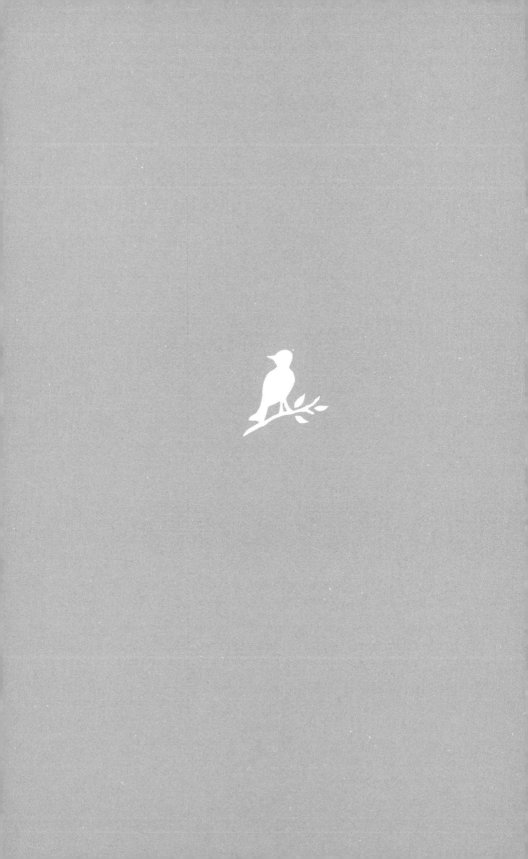

Let's Have Children

HAVING A CHILD IS ONE OF the most exhilarating and challenging life events you can ever experience. You're the lifeline to a new human being who is looking to you for everything from food to a clean diaper, fresh air, and entertainment. As a woman, the feeling of being that needed and loved—that you bring the sunshine to your child through your energy— is incredibly delightful. It's a whole new manifestation of love and the emergence of a new identity: mother.

Not everyone wants kids. Some couples feel fulfilled enough with each other and their interests, and that's fine! If you never want to have kids, already raised them, or wish to pawn them off on someone else, you can still glean insight from this chapter, since you will undoubtedly be around children, as well as the wretched people who have them. Joking aside, being familiar with the joys and struggles that arise might make you a better friend or aunt.

Having or not having children, how many children to have, and how they will be raised all has to be talked about ahead of time! Think how upset you'd be if you married someone and expected to have a big family with him and then found out that he only wants one child. Planning and communication are vital to the well-being of your relationship and the creation of your family.

Agree Ahead of Time . . .

Before you start trying for a baby, make sure that you and your partner have talked about parenting and agree on almost all fronts. Here are some topics to consider:

Waiting for the "Right" Time

Most kids would never have been born if their parents waited until it was the "perfect" time to have children. As much as we all want to have our ducks in a row by owning a home, having great jobs, and stowing fifty thousand dollars away in the bank, it rarely works that way. Financially it will probably never seem like quite the "right" time. The main consideration is: Do you and your husband have the sincere desire to bring a child into the world and raise him? Attitude is everything. When you both yearn to start a family, you will make it happen despite the obstacles—and there will always be obstacles.

Keep in mind that your life will change dramatically when you have a child. Gone are the days of grabbing a tiny purse and waltzing out the door. Women who don't have kids yet have no idea what it's like *not* to have so much me, me, I, I time. They have the freedom to spend a lot of hours sleeping in, lounging around, and going out, which can delude them into believing that's the way life always is. (Cue the laughter for the women with children.) The reality is that once you have a child, your needs definitely come second and maybe even third. And you have to be ever present mentally.

Pre-kids, you can freelance your days—like you decide to skip dinner and just have cheese, crackers, and wine. Enjoy that schedule while you can, because your life will need to become much more structured and family-centric once you have children. If you're not ready to let go of the carefree lifestyle you've enjoyed for years, it might not be the right time. The responsibility is enormous, so you have to really want it!

Another factor to consider is your relationship with your partner. Are you on strong terms and both prepared to have a baby? If yes, getting pregnant and giving birth can provide incredible bonding moments! But if you've been growing apart and things aren't working, there's nothing quite like a baby to make it all blow up in your face. It's a common misconception that having a child will help your marital problems. It won't. It will most likely make them worse. As such, be sure that this is truly the person you want to have children with.

When It's Not the Right Time

I would know. I had my daughter when I was eighteen. Is it a good idea to be a teenage mom? Probably not. Is it hard? Yes. Though Leisa was far from planned, I believe there are reasons why children are here, and I don't want to second-guess them. That being said, I think women should be free to make their own decisions about what's best for their health and lives.

I sometimes joke that I'm surprised Leisa is still alive. As a teenage mom, I was on my game, but because of my young age I was still learning how to manage my own life, let alone an infant's. I remember when Leisa found my vitamin bottle and swallowed a bunch of capsules. I had to have her stomach pumped. As you can imagine, the whole situation was incredibly upsetting and humbling. I made mistakes, but I kept finding my way, and I believe that's the process with any mother—regardless of age or other factors. Even when a pregnancy is unplanned and the timing is lousy, an oops baby will become your pride and joy. Leisa certainly became mine!

How Many to Have and How Far Apart?

Get in agreement with your partner on how many children you'd ideally like to have. I've found that a lot of men want big families and the women are like, what? No way! The guy could have grown up in a large family and hopes for that experience again, or maybe he didn't have a good relationship with his family and intends to create his own close-knit family now. On the other hand, the guy who says, "I don't care how many children we have" scares me because you can't have him checking out and leaving the childrearing up to you. His attitude and tax forms need to show that he cares very much! Before you get married, discuss your ideal family size and come to a compromise on a target number. He wants four; you want two; could you settle on three?

When you have one child and want another, figuring out when to have the second one can be tricky. The second child is usually easier than the first because you've been through the routines and know what to expect, but if baby #1 is still in diapers and breastfeeding, you might not feel ready to welcome baby #2. Some people, though, want to roll the first one into the next to get the baby stage over and done with. That's the intentional Irish-twin route.

I've known many women who were not ready to start on the next child, but their husbands were. A woman seeing that her hot, pre-pregnancy body has gotten stretched out and flabby might not like it when her husband says, "Hey, babe, let's have another one!" She thinks, I haven't even gotten back in shape yet and you want me to balloon up again? Or, I haven't slept through the night in months, but you think it's time for another baby? On the other hand, often the woman is ready and the man is not. Again, try to reach a compromise. When people love and care for one another, they can understand their mate's concerns and work out a mutually agreeable solution.

Let's say you think you're ready for the next child. Be honest with yourself. Can you handle your life well now? Is your hair standing on end and your husband quaking in the corner? What does the next year look like? Are you getting enough support to pull it off? Of course you should always talk to your doctor to find out if it's a safe or advisable time to try for another child.

Who Will Do What?

The days of the woman-only approach to raising children are over. They have gone the way of the milkman, who may or may not have fathered those children to begin with. In earlier generations childrearing was considered the female's realm and the guy's main responsibility was bringing home the money. Now it's common for both people to contribute to the financial well-being of the household, as well as the laundry and diaper changing. "We are getting pregnant" is the new norm, and I am all for it. I think couples should plan to share the responsibilities that come with having children and prepare for their new family by taking prenatal classes and reading parenting books together.

After all, it's a life adventure that you're embarking on, and you will need all hands on deck. You don't want the situation in which you tell your husband what you learned about breastfeeding as he's turning on the TV and replying, "Oh, that's cool," but you know he hasn't listened to a word you've said. That type of environment makes a pregnant woman feel very alone. The husband needs to be as involved as the wife—before and after the baby comes. In the past, men pretty much only listened to the woman talk about what was happening with the baby if the situation was drastic. It was a martini after work followed by an episode of *The Honeymooners*. Since no one will be time traveling back to the 1950s, it's best to plan on adopting the new way of doing things.

However, that's not to say that everything is split 50/50. It depends on the couple. If the woman stops working for a year or two to raise the child, then she might create a schedule with her husband in which he helps her with the baby for a couple of hours in the evenings. On the weekends he can contribute more time. As far as sleeping goes, one person can't be up all night with the baby daily. Take turns. Put him on baby duty one night; you take it the other.

You know me: I love plans! And the more you can plan ahead of time on who will do what and when, the smoother things will go once the baby actually arrives.

Church, School, Chores, and More

Will you raise your children with religion? Do you plan on sending them to public or private school? What types of chores will they have? It's important to talk about how you plan to raise your children. Childrearing differences can wreak havoc on a marriage and create confusing mixed messages in the family.

It's also important to come to agreement on how strict you're going to be with your kids before you actually have them. Though it will be a long time before they can talk (and talk back) and walk (and walk away), it's critical that you and your husband see eye to eye on how discipline and structure will be handled in the household. More on this shortly.

When the Baby Arrives . . .

It doesn't matter how much you have prepared for this baby. You could have read every book on parenting that's ever been written and listened to over one hundred mothers' advice, but nothing can prepare you for the whirlwind ahead. It is OTT: over the top.

You will be sleep deprived and frazzled and cow-like: heavy, awkward, and full of milk. At times, you will be completely overwhelmed by the energy this baby requires. And you will be bowled over by your love for this new life.

Nothing changes your lifestyle more suddenly or drastically than motherhood. You now have a tiny being who depends completely upon you. It will be strange to be wedded to a schedule that revolves around feeding and sleeping and pooping. You'll also be surprised by the amount of gear you schlep everywhere. Leaving the house will not be the simple task it used to be!

Despite the challenges—and there are many—children are a blessing who really make us go inside ourselves and reflect. When you become a mother, you learn that the things you thought were important, like how you look, are not. Your child takes the highest priority, and the "me" era comes to a screeching halt. I remember making sure that Leisa looked nicely put together with braided hair and cute shoes, yet I would only take fifteen minutes for myself to shower and dress. I didn't mind dashing out the door with wet hair and clothes that didn't match as long as Leisa was well cared for.

When you are responsible 24/7 for an infant, your priorities, relationships, and identity all shift. It happens quickly, which can be confusing and upsetting for many women who begin to ask themselves, "Who am I now?" You are a mother, which means that a new realm of existence has opened up for you. This is scary and splendid. You'll probably start thinking more deeply about your relationship with your own mother, your childhood, and how you want to be as a mother. Fathers go through a similar process and begin to see themselves as providers. Your identity as individuals gets reshaped into a family, and it's a beautiful transformation for both of you. It's like new leaves and branches growing on an already thriving tree.

But this is also a time of doubts and fears. You'll wonder whether you can adequately care for the baby's needs and if you're being a good mother. That's normal. After all, it's common to be afraid of unknowns, and motherhood is a big unknown for you!

As you prepare for this new phase as "Mom," take a deep breath and this general advice: You and your husband need to work out a system so that *each of you gets some alone time* while the other person is caring for the baby. During that time, squeeze a workout in, take a bath, read a book—whatever it is that you feel you need to do for your own health. To be a good caretaker, you have to take care of yourself. If you're a single parent, reach out to relatives and friends. Even a thirty-minute break will feel like a miracle. Mothers need time to recharge.

It's okay not to be perfect. Unless you're super vain, you will not perceive yourself as the world's best mom from day one. After all, you're new to it. You wouldn't expect someone to ace a new career in two weeks. Parenting is learning from mistakes, accepting that you're not perfect, and having a good attitude to face it another day—or hire a nanny.

New mothers get overwhelmed and worry that they're not making the right choices, which leads to a lot of second-guessing, but that all gets sorted out. There's no such thing as a perfect mother, and the sooner you realize that, the better off you'll be. Put a group of mothers in a room and one is feeding her child organic food; one is using regular food; one has a sleep schedule in place; one does not. Don't feel the need to compare yourself to other mothers. You and your baby will be just fine because what matters most are the love and support that the parents give a child.

Realize that your instincts will start to kick in. Eventually you'll know what a certain cry means and the best way to soothe your baby. It will come to you quickly because you don't want your child to be unhappy. You gain a different voice, skills, and a whole new way of interpreting yourself to a child. It's very rewarding. I loved it!

Soon you'll master carrying the baby, baby bag, and the stroller down the stairs and opening the door with so much balance you could have a plate propped on your head. You develop an ability to organize items quickly and to plan ahead to meet the needs of the baby. Your mind is always in a planning mode.

You develop this amazingly acute sense of hearing because you're always listening for a cry or a choke. Your days of sleeping soundly are over. You don't want to sleep like a rock because you want to stay in tune with what's going on with your child, and it's a pain in the ass because men sleep through everything!

Don't sweat the guilt trips. You want to be super mom, but occasionally you think longingly of those single, easy-breezy days! Then you wonder, what kind of mom am I to miss going to happy hour and movie dates when I have this marvelous child? You are just a normal mom. It's natural to need a baby break. After all, you are an adult who likes to have conversations that go beyond cooing noises. So leave the guilt to your mother-in-law, and cut yourself some slack. Once you get a little bit of distance from your baby, you'll be able to unwind, which will put you in a good mood. A good mood and new energy means a happy baby.

Save up. Having children is expensive! Between food, clothes, shelter, education, and health insurance, that wee little thing goes through cash like diapers! Do your best to set aside as much as you can afford for day-to-day necessities as well as long-term goals, like a college fund.

For your and your baby's health, it's important to stay calm. Have you ever seen a dog act nuts? It's usually because its owners act nuts, too. It's important to use techniques, like deep breathing and meditation, to stay tranquil and in harmony with your child. There will be times when you feel like you just can't take it, and that's quite normal. It's natural to get overwhelmed. What you'll notice, though, is that the baby will sense your frustration and become fussier. This can be a vicious cycle. Your stress becomes the baby's stress, which becomes your stress again. Here are a few ways to keep that stress from spreading:

Deep breathing (take a deep breath and hold it for ten seconds; repeat; your heart rate will drop)

Massage (loosen up those muscles and inhale the soothing scents of lavender or sandalwood)

Exercise (it will melt away the stress and get you back in shape; go for a fast walk or jog with the stroller so that the baby gets some fresh air, too)

Yoga (exercise + relaxation = zen mom)

Meditation (clear away the mental clutter and worry)

Join a friend for some baby-free fun (you need an adult break from time to time!)

If you have a particularly colicky or difficult baby and just don't know how you can keep going, remember this: The baby phase only lasts twelve months. Then it's over and pretty soon you have teenagers—oh, the horror! Seriously, as much as you may want the sleepless nights to end, it will also mean the end of all the exciting firsts (smile, laugh, sitting up). Everything passes, so enjoy the good parts and don't agonize over the bad parts. Soon life will take you and your child to a new phase.

Beyond the Cradle

Every little step that your child takes toward the next milestone also brings her closer to independence. You want your baby to grow and walk and become a kindergartener who reads who becomes a third grader who plays the piano and so forth. But it's bittersweet, because each accomplishment means that your little one needs you less and less and is becoming older and older.

Eventually you go from controlling when your children eat and sleep to witnessing them become mini adults with opinions and unique characteristics. The fourteen-to-eighteen-year age bracket can be very tough. You feel like you've gone to the *Twilight Zone* with your children. Now you're not hip or with it in their eyes. It's like the woman at the grocery store who asked me the other day if I needed help out to the car. I told her I'd look her up in twenty years, but I don't need any help now. Well, kids eventually get that same attitude. They don't think they need you anymore, but they don't make good decisions.

They'll stay up all night playing video games, for instance, if allowed to. You can take measures to deal with the situation, like taking away the video games and grounding them, but they are starting to express who they want to be, so it's an ongoing challenge. When they were seven, you thought they were going to be a certain kind of child, like an athlete or musician, but now they don't like sports or instruments at all. When you don't identify with the way they're behaving, parenting becomes really difficult. How do you deal with those feelings of frustration? You drink a lot and carry a big stick.

Everyone finds his or her way, but you're worried your kid is going to find his way to a mirror lined with cocaine or a tattoo parlor. You have to try to lead by example. If you tell your kid not to drink, but you're slamming down the cocktails every night, she or he might not take you seriously. You have got to be someone who your kids think is grounded and respectable. Kids are looking for stability. They're looking for structure and discipline. The parents who don't think that's the case are incorrect. Kids want to be told, "This is what time you go to bed," though they might not like it that very moment.

Some parents want to be their kids' best friends, and that's a mistake. I once did a seminar in which I asked people, "How many of you feared your parents?" Then I asked, "How many of you to this day love your parents?" The same people raised their hands. Many people in my generation grew up fearing their parents. As a result (even though they seemed to have forgotten that they still loved their parents despite the strict upbringing), they decided to approach parenting differently and to take the easy, anything-goes road with their own children. Kids want boundaries. I am not for the parents who let their children misbehave without consequences or who give false threats and don't follow through.

Along those lines, don't fall into the good cop/bad cop trap. If the child gets a no from mom, but dad says yes, the lesson the child takes away is "just ask dad." Kids should know that their parents are a united front, not a democracy in which the child gets a vote and learns how to lobby and make side deals. I can't tell you how many people have told me that it drives them crazy how their spouse always has to be the nice one, which means they're always the bad one. They feel undermined and disliked, because kids gravitate toward the more lenient parent. Later in life children will realize that the "no" parent really cared about them rather than just wanting to please them or not deal with them. Discipline is much easier to enforce if you both support each other's decisions and are in agreement about what the rules are and the consequences for breaking them.

It's all about balance. You have to discipline children, but also let them be who they are. The best thing you can do is make your children feel loved and acknowledged. Children know when your attention is sincere and that you're listening to them and are a part of their world. They can sense when they're not being seen or heard, as can adults and pets. Being there, being consistent, and doing what you think is best will help you through the sometimes temperamental teen years.

Blending Families

Having and raising children doesn't always follow a cookie-cutter pattern. Many people get divorced, remarry, and blend their families together. Or they might have never been married to begin with, and they have a child. Let's say that he's got a five-year-old, you have a seven-year-old, and you're now going to raise them together in the same household and possibly have a new baby together. Creating a mixed-family environment can work out wonderfully, but it's not without its challenges.

"Problem children" are a common complaint from my clients and a reason why I acquire new business. Recently, for one of my clients I found a female match who was available after she'd broken up with a man she'd lived with for two years because she couldn't stand his children's behavior. They were difficult teenagers who often got in trouble. One of them was arrested multiple times. It wasn't a situation that she wanted in her life. The ex-boyfriend is a solid guy who acquired majority custody, and he's trying to be strict and maintain order, but it just wasn't working out and she didn't have the patience to see where it all went.

Many matchmaking clients have told me that they're looking for a partner either with no children or grown children. No one has ever said to me, "I would love to find someone who has teenagers." But misery loves company, so if you both have teens you've got a shot at finding a love connection. He'll think "You've got bad kids; I've got bad kids. I think we should put all of our bad kids together and be the good, the bad, and the ugly." I am just kidding, of course, and I truly believe that if you try hard enough, the right situation will manifest itself. However, if you're a single mom and your children have been acting bratty or defiant, you're going to need to get a handle on that if you want to successfully incorporate a new partner into the fold.

As I said before, don't introduce a new boyfriend to your children right away. I've seen it really upset kids who kept meeting all these different people and never witnessing any of them sticking around for longer than a few months. Be in a very significant relationship before you introduce a child to a boyfriend.

Your children might be slow to warm to the new guy. Give them time to adjust, and communicate openly with them. If your children are outright rude, you need to talk to them. It's up to the parent to say, "You're making it difficult for me to find and keep love in my relationships because you are an extension of me and you're not being nice. If in fact you want me to find someone and further our happiness as a family, then I am asking you to give Ken a chance." You might need to go to counseling as a family to work through the transition. It's not easy, and generally the older the children are (unless they're grown and out of the house), the harder it is. But it's not impossible, and there's no reason to throw up a white flag and surrender to solo-dom.

You deserve love. Your children deserve love. You new partner or partner-to-be deserves love. And just because your new boyfriend isn't your child's biological father does not mean that your child won't grow to love him as if he were. Human beings are capable of so much love and bonding. The family possibilities are limitless if you're willing to work for them. You can have new children together, combine families Brady-Bunch style, or maybe one of you has children and the other doesn't and that is a big enough family for both of you.

The key is just making sure that each child feels important. If you have a daughter and want to have a baby with a new dad, tell your daughter, "We're a family and we're all having this baby together and you are going to help us with the baby. Isn't it exciting that you're going to have a sister or brother to play with now?" Kids will accept a new role as long as they feel included and loved.

This wraps up child chat: zero to eighteen in just one chapter! Obviously having and raising children is a broad topic, but for the purposes of this book I am choosing to look at it as one major step along the relationship cycle. It might be a step you are heading to for the first time, returning to with a new spouse, skipping with a "good riddance," or re-evaluating as you become a grandmother or aunt. Nonetheless it's time to move on to a not-so-cheery subject . . .

Leave or Stay?

TO STAY OR NOT TO STAY? That can be one of the hardest questions in life to answer. You've put time and energy into a relationship that now seems like a train that's run out of steam. The excitement that powered the train is gone, and you don't see a way forward. Or, maybe there's enough love and respect to fall back on that re-energizes the relationship and keeps it moving down the track. It really just depends on the two people and the situation they find themselves in.

As I've said before, you're in your own movie. You're watching it and need to decide if it will play out well or if it's time for a new script. Does a handsome train robber come around and whisk you away? Do you jump off the train and run to the next town, where you become the first female sheriff? Do you push Mr. Wrong off the train and then pretend like nothing happened? (That's taking "dumping" to the extreme, and I don't recommend it!)

Whether it's living together, long term, short term, married, or any other kind of relationship, you commit and work on things until you don't see a way forward. It is much better to release someone to a new beginning and a better match than to wear each other down into miserable living graves. Though zombie action films are popular, don't let your movie turn that way!

One person's trash is another person's treasure. You don't want to make your partner wrong for who he is or what he does. Maybe his goodness can't shine through with you anymore, or yours can't shine through with him. It's okay to say this isn't working. It's okay to end it. There are many "someones" out there for everyone; what drives you crazy might delight another person. Give each other the blessing of a fresh start.

However, sometimes things happen in a relationship that hurt and frustrate you, but they aren't deal-breakers. They can be addressed, learned from, and fixed. Sometimes it takes work to get the train back on the track, and sometimes you'd rather run off with the conductor.

In this chapter we'll take a look at what to do when you hit a snag and how you know when to go versus when to stay. It's like the Kenny Rogers' song, "You got to know when to hold 'em, know when to fold 'em, know when to walk away and know when to run."

Signs That It's Time to Leave

Everyone has a breaking point. You can keep doing something and doing something and all of a sudden you can't do it anymore. You've lost respect for the other person, and you don't see him taking any action to improve the situation, and you just know you're done.

I struggled with my then-husband for years and years with the same-old situation of him being underemployed and after awhile it was like, oh my God, how is this ever going to end? I kept trying to be optimistic and make recommendations of what he could do for work, and pretty soon it was more my dream than his. He was really comfortable taking his sweet time to figure out what he wanted. Money was not a high priority for him. Suffocation set in, and I started to get panic attacks. I was on a rat wheel, financially supporting us and handling all the bills and IRS payments. I didn't need him to be the breadwinner; I just wanted him to meet me halfway.

He was (and is) a very good-looking guy, but after a while that wasn't enough. Financial issues began to diminish the attraction. Instead of being turned on when seeing him strutting around in his boxers, I wanted his legs to be covered in trousers and off at work making money.

I had to end it for both of us to go on. You might wonder, "Why didn't you give him more time to prove himself?" Well, when you quit believing in the person you're with it's very hard to go another day together. You have to trust in a person's ability to do right by you and the relationship; if you don't, it's almost impossible to move forward. We divorced after ten years of marriage, and he found a fabulous connection for himself and a lifestyle that suits him much better. And I found a better match and lifestyle for myself. That is the upside of divorce and breakups.

Believe me, there are plenty of signals that will tell you when it's time to walk, and I'm not talking about the green man at crosswalks. You will see obvious signs that the relationship has major flaws. It's just a question of whether you pay attention to them or rationalize them away.

Here are common indicators (deal breakers) that you should move on:

- A bad behavior, whether it's cheating, abuse, drinking, unemployment, general disrespect, or anything else that strongly affects you and the relationship, becomes a habit that you don't believe will ever end.

- The resentment gets so strong that you can't move forward. There are no pieces you can pick up. There is no love or respect to fall back on.

- Whenever there is any kind of physical abuse, leave. Run. You deserve better. Don't put up with emotional abuse either. Women need to be strong and to love and believe in themselves and a better future.

- You have a general sense that it's a lack of life you're living, and you can't find anything you enjoy anymore about the relationship.

- When your partner shows no effort to change behaviors that are causing problems and takes the attitude of, oh well, we can just go down like the Titanic, then there's no point in hoping for a rescue boat. Without a willingness to talk about what's wrong or a plan for how to fix it, you have no options. A big thing for me is seeing that the person is trying. Everything is done in energy and timeframes.

♦ The relationship starts affecting your health. Like many self-help practitioners, I believe that built-up resentment and other stressful emotions lead to illness. The body shuts down and doesn't function well. Little bits and pieces of tearing your heart out and the emotional pain you suffer can become a physical malady. Pay attention to your health—I see girls whose health is often falling apart and it coincides completely with what's going on in their relationships—and get out of any relationship that has a consistently harmful effect on it.

♦ If the relationship weighs you down more often than it picks you up, then heed the red flag waving right in your face. There are normal stresses that you have to handle in life (a rebellious teenager, your husband getting laid off) and those will test your character, but the relationship itself shouldn't crush your spirits. A person who is a good match for you makes you feel safe, secure, loved, and respected. He is self-sufficient, competent, and responsible. Your partner should charge your batteries, not suck the life out of you. When you find yourself with a dead battery in a relationship, leave the relationship to find the jump you need, whether it's jumping someone's bones or jumping off a cliff with a parasail on your back.

Again, when things aren't working well, there are obvious signs. If you find yourself wondering how these problems are going to end, you've got to shake yourself and ask, "Is this really what I deserve? Is this it? Am I going to subject myself to this kind of a life?" If you're not a fan of prison, don't do it. People cling to their bad relationships. It's like having stacks of clothes you'll never wear in your closet; there comes a time when you have to cleanse. You have to face the truth that the relationship is not working and accept that it's time to end it.

Keep in mind that ending a relationship releases two people to a new beginning. Most of the time both people grow from their experience and find better matches. In our society, we accept the idea of learning from mistakes and starting anew in various capacities, yet when it comes to relationships there is still a lot of negativity around divorce. That's unfortunate and ridiculous, because obviously a practice that is so common (about half of marriages end in divorce) shows us that marriage is a difficult endeavor that we frequently can't sustain over time. I often use the word "release" instead of "divorce" because I believe we have to be more positive and understanding about a process that's as ordinary and messy as dirt.

Why Women Stay When They Should Run

It can take a life-threatening situation or tragedy for the alert light to go off. Life and time are immeasurably valuable. Are you happy? Is this relationship going nowhere? Do you want to finish off the rest of your life being miserable? There's always another person out there who will treat you like a prize. No one needs to settle for less. Women in particular hold on and hold on when their gut is telling them to let go.

Why? It's often about money and fear. As my close friend Linda says, "Money doesn't make you happy. It just makes life easier." I couldn't agree more. I divorced at age 51. I had about $540 left in my bank account, my only money in the whole world. I withdrew five one-hundred-dollar bills, went over to my friends' house, and laid the bills on the table. I said, "Well, this is it. This is what I have left." They were very concerned and asked, "Are you okay?" I said, "I'll be fine." I've never had a fear of being broke. I've always been confident that I could find a way to make money. At that time, my overhead (between my business and personal finances) ran about $10,000 a month. Some people might have panicked. I told myself that I had new clients coming in and that I'd make it work, and I did.

I've had it all—the Porsche Carrera and the financial planner and luxurious vacations—and I've been stripped of it all, too. You can't get too attached to "stuff." Fear and despair will kill your spirit. In difficult situations like this, I ask myself: What do I need to do to control my life?

I believe there's a manual for everything and that self-confidence will carry me forward.

Women worry that as a result of divorce they'll lose everything: the house, the country-club membership, the car, the mutual friends, and so forth. Well guess what? The long-term stress from staying in a bad relationship is like living with a bomb inside your body that's about to go off. You're better off to take a new approach to life than stick with one that's slowly killing you.

In addition to financial fears, many women stay in bad relationships because they fear that they'll never find love again. As I've said before, how much love we've collected at the end of our lives determines the kind of life we've lived. There is no limit to love; it does not exist solely in one relationship. If you love yourself, you will find love in the world. Men who are jerks brainwash women into thinking, look at you. How are you going to do better than me? Don't heed those messages! They aren't true.

People can get so wrapped up in their relationships that they can't see the situation for what it really is and why they should leave. I was saddened by a woman named Sarah, who recently told me about her sexless marriage. Sarah said that after she got pregnant with her son, who is now twenty-one years old, her husband never had sex with her again. He got very angry about her getting pregnant and has apparently never forgiven her. Sarah is a beautiful woman and they are both highly-paid professionals with what one would consider a lot of options. She has stayed with him only because, in her opinion, divorce screws up children. (I will address the subject of children and divorce in the next chapter.) They've played house for the so-called benefit of their son, who ironically is very close to his father. No wonder Sarah has a hot trainer! I couldn't imagine living that way (even with a studly trainer as eye candy), but I'd be a liar if I said Sarah's case is a rarity. Women (and men) stay decades too long in broken relationships.

Time goes very quickly and we all hate to throw in the towel. In some cases, we stay because we know the problems we've agreed to instead of trying on someone else's problems, which are unknowns. But I say, why fear the unknown when the known makes you sad and frustrated? Also keep in mind that a good relationship should build your self-esteem. If you're feeling bad about yourself, that's probably a sign that your partner isn't cherishing you or that the two of you just can't fulfill each other's needs anymore.

My advice is to always be prepared for the next step in life so that if your relationship goes south, you can move on quickly and won't need two years to pull your health, finances, and self-esteem together.

Lastly, I believe in general that women start and end relationships. Even though in divorce court, for example, it appears on paper that the guy left his wife for another woman, in truth the wife left the husband a long time before that. Probably somewhere along the line, the communication between the two of them stopped. She really wanted the relationship to be over so she pushed him away, he acted out, and that gave her the reason that she was looking for to justify calling it quits. Tag; you're it. I know this isn't always the case, but I use this hypothetical example as a way of saying, "Women, listen up. You need to understand your role in a relationship's continuation or end. You have a lot more power than you may believe."

Stress Tests

What, then, are situations that will test your relationship and either send it plunging over the ledge or strengthen it for years to come?

People ask me what the number-one takedown in a relationship is. Is it lack of love, money, or attention? To me it's lifestyle. Money will never override lifestyle; you cannot buy lifestyle. It is the key to togetherness. People need to enjoy some of the same activities and have like-minded ideas of how to spend their free time together.

Money is also hugely influential on relationships. Many a divorce has been filed over financial troubles. Struggling to pay for groceries and rent doesn't help love, and financial difficulties lead to animosity. I've seen situations in which the woman no longer feels like the sex kitten in the bedroom because she has to be the whistleblower on what's going on with their money and investments. She's lost her femininity in the realm of the relationship after wearing the pants for too long and constantly making tough decisions for the two of them. That can work fine when the woman has the better business sense and doesn't mind being the anchor. But anytime there is resentment about what you have to do for another person, the relationship suffers.

You can get to a point, like one couple I know, when you're having heated arguments about subjects as insignificant as how many paper towels you're going through in a week's time. There wasn't a paper towel in the world that could absorb that much bile. I've said it before and I'll say it again: money is a major relationship takedown, so as much as you possibly can, get your financial affairs in order before you get married.

Arguments of any kind that don't lead to resolutions take their toll on a relationship. The arguing stems from not understanding or appreciating each other's views of reality. You have to really comprehend and respect how your partner sees the world. If you can't relate to each other or compromise, you're in for a rocky ride. Also, when one person thinks that too much responsibility has been placed on him or her, irritation and discontent will ensue, and they don't tango well with romance.

Sometimes your partner doesn't grow into the person you feel you need in your life. My friend Cathy married her first husband when they were both twenty. As time went on, she wanted him to be more ambitious, driven, and stronger; in other words, she wanted a type A. But that wasn't his nature. It can be a challenge when, after marrying young, your spouse doesn't evolve in the way you want him to. Let's face it: our needs change and often in unexpected ways. Cathy left him and found the driven partner she wanted, and he married someone who loved him for who he was.

It breaks my heart when I meet couples whose relationship struggles are a result of addiction. Addiction troubles overtax a relationship and need to be resolved for the relationship to function. Anything you put a higher priority on than your family and take to excess, whether it's food, drugs, alcohol, porn, or something else, causes deep imbalance. For instance, a client named Jessica previously married a man who developed a workout addiction and spent up to four hours in the gym daily. That caused a lot of stress, and they eventually separated. My friend Rebecca married a guy who turned out to be a closet drinker. She had no idea before marrying Hank that he had a problem. He refused to take control of his addiction or change his ways, so she divorced him, but Rebecca was devastated about it.

Unlike addiction, sexual problems put strain on relationships but can usually be worked through. As mentioned before, a common problem is that the guy wants sex more frequently than the woman. To resolve it, normally one or the other has to give in a little, which means either he has to accept less nooky or she has to put her game face on more often. That's usually a fairly easy compromise to reach. If the problem is of a physical nature, we live in the pharmaceutical age and can quickly address it in the form of Viagra, for example. Voilà instant hardness.

On the subject of sex, infidelity really tests the waters, but it doesn't always spell the end. In my experience, most of the time couples stay together after an instance of cheating. If they sit down and go over why it happened, they gain insight into their relationship and work through the issues. Maybe the man realizes that he's been wrapped up in his business and hasn't paid his wife enough attention, which resulted in her seeking attention elsewhere, or maybe she sees that she's withdrawn too much from her husband and has started living a separate life. Contrary to what many people assume, infidelity has nothing to do with how much sex the couple is having. And despite the gender stereotype of the man being the one who runs around on his poor unsuspecting wife, research and my own observations have shown that women are often the ones who cheat. In other words, it's not just men who stray.

Depending on a person's situation and personality, one time of cheating can be one too many, and he or she is out the door. It's all about reacting in the way that feels right to you. You should only stay if you want to and can get back on track together and let go of the bitterness. Some people remain but then fall into a dysfunctional pattern of constantly punishing the person who cheated in small and large ways. That won't work over time and will just make both people miserable.

It's a different scenario altogether when the cheating becomes a habit. The second time it's not a mistake; it's a repeated behavior that is harder to forgive because the person can't claim it was a one-time lapse in judgment that won't happen again. In cases of serial cheating, I've probably seen just as many people stay as go. Unfortunately, many women internalize their husbands' cheating. They think, it must have happened because I'm not good-looking enough. They start getting facelifts and liposuction and work out obsessively. These women make their husbands' infidelity their own problem, instead of holding the men accountable. It becomes a way of life. Ladies, if you allow yourself to live with a cheater and you keep putting up with it, then you have low self-esteem and you have a problem, too, not just the cheater. You can't send people the message that they can disrespect or mistreat you, because they will make a habit of it, which isn't healthy for either of you. I would know.

My ex-husband Rick, the professional baseball player, enjoyed many one-night stands while on the road. Now, did I believe at the time that he was falling in love with any of these women or thinking of leaving me? No, I really didn't. I thought of them as fleeting physical connections—part of a game that he was playing in his personal life as well as on the field. He loved the attention. I used to talk to other baseball wives who didn't give a darn about any of the fooling around. Their attitude was my husband always comes back to me, so who cares? Well, that may have worked for them, but on a deeper level it mattered to me.

As women we try to be strong and put on a proud face, but holding that kind of pain inside is destructive. Rick's other problems escalated the tension and he became abusive. That's why I eventually left him, but I shouldn't have put up with any of his misbehavior for as long as I did. I stayed too long, and I fault myself for that. I thought he would get help and get better, but in the end my only option was to get out. A lesson I would like everyone to learn from this book is that there are always options! You are never stuck and can always take action to improve or leave a relationship.

Reasons to Stay

Relationships can be exasperating. They're not all champagne and bouquets, but problems don't have to predict disaster. Many conflicts can be dealt with, and the first step is always communication.

Couples usually are together because they love each other. They don't intentionally want to cause each other pain. So, for example, if you don't speak up about what's bothering you, your husband might not realize that anything's wrong. Never underestimate the potential cluelessness of a man! I can't tell you how many men are shocked when their wives announce that they want a divorce. The men didn't see it coming because their wives rarely communicated about the behaviors that bothered them. Many times women talk to their friends and family instead of their husbands. I could name many of my girlfriends who don't say anything directly to their husbands, who are driving them crazy. Silence will solve nothing!

Anything can become a bad habit. The key is nipping in the bud any behavior you see that isn't working for you before it causes a lot of damage. When something's bothering you, just say it. Don't hint, nag, play passive-aggressive, or give him the long version. Cut to the chase. "I'm really unhappy with what we do during the week. I would love to go for walks at night and have date-night once a week." Then see what he says. He'll probably be willing to change things. If you, however, say to him, "I can't believe you watch TV every night! Doesn't this life bore you to tears? I didn't realize you were this boring when I married you," then you're asking for trouble. Never put a guy on the defensive unless you want a big blowout—and I'm not talking about a Macy's sale.

Try to talk about, modify, and reassess behaviors that are causing relationship strain. It can help to bring in a third party, like a financial planner (if that's the area of conflict) or a counselor or psychologist. If your partner refuses to work on things and gives you the my-way-or-the-highway attitude, that is not good and you should explore what the highway has to offer. Whether the problem is flirtation, financial irresponsibility, irritating in-laws, or anything else, you have to keep everything in check to prevent matters from snowballing into irreconcilable differences. It's like being a lifetime monitor; you have to constantly assess how everything's going.

I think that every week couples should sit down together and ask, "How are we doing? Is there anything that you need from me that you're not getting? Is there anything I could be doing to make our life together happier?" Staying on top of whatever threatens to take your relationship off course is a proactive way to deal with problems before they become deal breakers. Too often women try to overdo pleasing men to avoid conflict, but it backfires. The women end up resenting their partners and suffering in silence.

It can be the littlest thing that, in time, sets you off. One woman I know who works full-time has a husband who insists that she cook him a hearty breakfast three times a week. She hates it, but she's been doing it consistently for years and years. Somewhere along the line that became a very bad habit that she needs to address. He might think she loves doing it; next thing he knows he's going to find rat poison on his fried egg.

When your partner's actions begin to needle you, ask yourself: Why did I fall in love with this person? What does he bring to my life? Go back to his list of strengths. Often you can get a handle on the problem and realize you're getting your back up about a minor issue and that your husband is a wonderful guy. Focus on what you share together in energy, personality, and lifestyle.

Unfortunately, however, that ten percent of the person that goes bad in a relationship can be what takes you down. That ten percent can taint the other ninety percent to the extent that you just can't see an end in sight. If that's not the case, think of your husband's talents and capitalize on them. What does he do that is exceptional? For instance, an acquaintance Jocelyn said to me recently, "I don't know how you get your husband to cook dinner for you like that several times a week." Truthfully, I don't get my husband to do anything. He loves to cook, and I praise him for it, which makes him feel good and reinforces the behavior. There are many special gifts that each of us possesses that go ignored or underutilized. If there is life left in your relationship, find it and foster it so that you can feel the sparks again.

Speaking of sparks, it's common for people, especially women, to get bored after many years in a marriage. If you asked couples who have been married for twenty years how many weekends out of a month they're bored, it would be a scary seminar. Though it's normal to feel blah and not have that tingly, in-love sensation all the time, I don't think normal needs to stay in place for very long. Sometimes we need to change things up. You could be the one who always executes the change while the other person is fine with the way things are, but that doesn't matter. Put your ego aside and take charge of it and do what you can to stimulate newness. Being unable to shake the blahs might mean that you need couples therapy. Be in it; understand it; don't be impatient, but don't stay in the down cycle too long. Generate excitement as we talked about in chapter eleven.

Men are attached to patterns that work for them. For instance, why did I even bother to ask my husband today what flight he was taking? He's always on the 12:05 p.m. plane to Vegas. Things that are different make men skittish. Why? Because they're control freaks. Men like to control their environments. So women, listen up. If you want something that your husband did for you that was out of the box, like taking you shopping in Beverly Hills or having a picnic on the beach together, to happen again, then you'd better go into overdrive with the praise. I'm not kidding you. Give your husband more adoration than you could ever imagine because men love it. You might think, no, my husband is not like that; baloney, lady! But I'll tell you that men love knowing they did something to make you happy, and they'll repeat the action because they'll remember the benefits.

You can probably count on one hand what men are: their jobs, their clicker, and their golf games, running, and once-a-year fishing trips. What are women? We've got about thirty hands. With men, it's basic, so you need to work on cultivating that excitement. Boredom can just be a natural tendency, and you need to fight it every step of the way to keep your relationship fresh as spring rain.

Lastly, I don't believe that the best relationships are two people hooked at the hip 24/7. You can find a lot of the stimulation you're looking for in friendships, family, jobs, hobbies, sports, and volunteer work. Don't think of your husband or partner as being your whole world. Design a relationship that works for both of you. I know married couples who live in separate homes during the week and only spend the weekend together. That's fine as long as it's mutually desirable. I truly believe when there's respect and love in the relationship that women can get anything they want if they take the right approach.

For those of you who are in the difficult position of questioning whether to stay in your current relationship or leave, there's an exercise in the back of the book on page 198 that helps you to weigh the reasons for and against splitting up.

In the next chapter, we'll look at what to do if you've made the decision to definitely end a relationship. Leaving is hard, but it's a necessary means to living your life by the philosophy of next and never stuck. Onwards and upwards!

CHAPTER
14

Sometimes It's Not Meant to Be Forever, and That's Okay

You should never feel like your life is over because your relationship is. You're still breathing. Pinch yourself; it'll hurt. That being said, I know how sad and difficult ending a relationship can be. It's important to keep in mind, however, that there were reasons why the relationship dissolved, and staying with those problems still in play would be much worse than the pain of separation.

What is the difference between a breakup and a divorce? Paperwork and money. In my opinion, a breakup is as hard as a divorce, especially if you've loved someone a long time. A piece of paper has nothing to do with a broken heart. There's still an emotional trail of sadness that exists beyond the law and the division of assets. This chapter looks at the best way to end a relationship (regardless of whether it's a divorce or other type of breakup), how to process the change afterwards, and how to move on.

As I've said before, when you end a relationship it always seems to work out better for both of you. In the immediate aftermath, you don't see it because you're hurting and stressed and resemble an actress in a Cymbalta ad. But over time you get clearer on what didn't work for you and why, which gives you a better idea of what to look for moving forward, because you are going to enter into another relationship after this! You're not going to die from this heartache; it's not life threatening. You will get up off the well-worn couch, throw the soggy Kleenex away, dab your teary eyes, and find another person to love you. Your ex will also find happiness—unless of course you don't want him to. Then we'll just pretend that he ends up with erectile dysfunction or terrible breath that keeps the ladies away.

The Do's and Don'ts of Telling Him It's Over

Generally, people don't decide in a year's time that they want a divorce. If I were a gambling woman, I would bet that the average person thinks about getting a divorce for about five years before actually doing it. Though in unmarried relationships people might mull over the decision to leave or stay for less time, it's still a process that often takes many months or even years. Relationship problems build and build. One domino topples another, which topples another. By the time you decide to divorce or break up with someone, most likely it's been so bad for so long that you just can't take it anymore. If you're not ready but you've been unhappy for a long time, ask yourself whether you are needlessly second-guessing. Vacillation is a waste of time. Make a decision to stay or go. Don't sit on the fence for too long. It's not fair to you or your partner.

If you decide to end a relationship, what should you do and say? First, make a plan to speak lovingly to your husband/boyfriend in a private, comfortable place such as your home. Once that's arranged and you're seated together, express your whole heart and soul about what's not working for you and why you can no longer see yourself continuing in the relationship. Don't make it about the other person or blame him for your unhappiness. For example, if he's a cold, unaffectionate type who's always working, you could say, "I feel really lonely and want close companionship and socially active weekends." Don't say, "You're a frigid prick who never makes time for me." He can figure it out by reading between the lines if he wants to!

Whatever you do, as I've advised before, don't say, "I don't love you anymore." That is hurtful, unnecessary, and often just plain untrue. If you loved a person at one point, you will probably continue to love him even if it's in a toned-down way. It's the classic case of loving someone but not feeling in love or compatible anymore. Even if your boyfriend cheated on you every day for a year and you can't stand him now, don't attack him with the I-don't-love-you sling. Tell him that you deserve to be treated with more respect and less exposure to STDs.

In my opinion, the optimal result of a divorce or breakup is for two people who spent that much time together to walk away as friends. I don't mean friends as in close buddies who meet for happy hour every Tuesday—more the idea of being civil and caring towards each other. You were friends to begin with and you shared part of your lives together, so why after you part ways would you not speak to each other in public? When you are considerate and mature enough to end things with respect and not with personal attacks, then you can be amicable with an ex. It might not happen at first, but the best of the best will work through the difficult feelings and keep blame and bitterness at bay. I also think that when you end a relationship on friendly terms, finding love again becomes easier. More on that shortly.

The Blindside Potential

Unfortunately for some men, they don't get any kind of a heads up that their wives are unhappy, so they're sitting at their desk one day and all of a sudden get served divorce papers. It's like shock therapy. Because those women are frightened of the potential drama of the I-can't-do-this-anymore interaction, they run straight to a lawyer and handle it all from a distance. I don't agree with that approach at all.

Now, even if you don't blindside your husband with divorce papers, he will still most likely be dumbfounded when you tell him you want to leave. He might say, "What can I do to keep you from making this decision? Do you want a separation instead? Maybe we shouldn't do this so fast. Can we work this out?" If a man really loves a woman, he'll fight to keep her. If there's no fight, then you can count your lucky stars that you made the right decision.

I would say most of the time men try to keep the marriage going because men, even if they're cheating on their wives, will try to have their cake and eat it too. They will try to exploit as many options as possible. If you keep putting up with their affairs, for example, they'll keep having them. I don't know of too many relationships in which the guy pulled the plug. Women usually are the ones who exit. If your husband or boyfriend wants to give things another chance, that's up to you to decide. If you are fed up with the relationship and can't imagine going another day in it, then don't. But after voicing your concerns, if you feel like there is something redeemable that's worth fighting for, then give it a chance. Be honest with yourself. Only you know.

Your Initial Reaction

Once a woman ends a relationship that's been dragging on in an unsatisfactory way, she often feels a great sense of relief. She's now empowered to make decisions that will send her life in a new direction, which can be welcoming after years of feeling stuck. With a divorce, the process can stretch on for a year or much longer if arguments over money or children ensue, which means that sense of relief might take a while to set in. A divorce is one of the rare cases when it's nice not to have money because no cash or assets means there are no financial considerations to bicker about! Regardless, even though a year sounds like a long time, it most likely will fly by.

Some people might say, Barbara, you're full of it. After a divorce you feel lonely, depressed, distraught, and can't even imagine what you're going to do next. I realize that many people have felt that way even when they knew they were making the right decision. But you can get through fear and sadness to enjoy a sense of relief when the process has been completed and you've started to move on. That closure allows you to take the next step, meet the next person, find the next place to live, and so forth. Next to the nth degree!

Be Positive and Look Ahead

After a divorce or breakup, it's important to tell yourself how much you love yourself. Realize there are no guarantees that relationships will last forever, and that's okay. Don't be hard on yourself because a relationship ended. In order to move forward, you have to love and take care of *you*.

Your health is first and foremost. You're never going to be good to yourself or anyone else if you don't take care of your health.

Secondly, keep going. Keep moving. Stay in motion. Never look back. A handful of women after becoming single think they want to go back to their ex-husbands to see if they made the right decision. After divorcing someone, ninety-five percent of the time going back for a second round won't work. There's a reason you left. There was a reason you were miserable. Don't lose sight of that. It's all about decisions. Keep running like Forrest Gump; eventually you're going to stop when you find that next life wherever and however it's going to be.

My Leaving Story (Well, One of Them)

I was crushed and angry after my first divorce because I watched all that I'd loved and worked for over the course of seventeen years go up in smoke. It was an ugly end to what had been at one time a beautiful relationship of fun, family, limelight, and adventure. The divorce was a big crash for me, and I think with every low you need to create a high. Though I had a lot of friends in Arizona, they were all married and I didn't want to be a third wheel replaying the past in an unsatisfying way, so I set my sights on San Diego in September of 1984. We used to go there in the summer to escape the Arizona heat and now that I had a new kind of heat to escape, San Diego seemed like just the right refuge.

After packing up my belongings, my dream home, a 4,600-square-foot Spanish-style house with a four-car garage that sold for a wash, was stripped down to bare walls and phone jacks. I looked around and thought, well, that's that. I deposited my divorce settlement check of about $100,000—not much when you consider the kind of baseball career Rick had. Then I put my English sheepdog, Anaka, in the passenger seat of my car and had a moving truck follow me to San Diego. I didn't have a place to rent or purchase waiting for me. I was winging it!

Six hours of driving later, the moving van and I arrived in the village of La Jolla (a gorgeous oceanfront area of San Diego). I saw a realtor's sign, parked, walked quickly into the office, and announced that I was looking for a place to rent by the beach. I wanted to sign a two-year lease that day, as well as pay the entire amount up front. The realtor looked at me like I was crazy and inquired if I was serious. She soon verified that I was when I signed for the second place she showed me, a 1,500-square-foot cottage with a deck on Palomar Street near Windansea beach. I paid by check for two years and had the moving truck unload my items. That night I passed out on top of the packing boxes.

I went from owning a massive designer home to renting a tiny cottage with French doors near the water. Stuff is stuff, and less is more. It's all about recreating energy around you. I knew San Diego would be good energy. I wanted to breathe—to start completely over. For some people, it makes more sense to stay in a place of comfort where your family and friends are. It all depends on your personality as well as your situation. The important thing is to trust your heart and intuition and make the necessary changes.

I was in my mid-thirties and wanted everything to be new. I would sit in the breakfast nook and look out at the ocean. The feeling of being single set in on me. Slowly, the layers of stress and confusion melted away. I accepted the loss and that all the rugs had been pulled out from under me and embraced the idea of starting over.

Anaka, my sheepdog, played a huge part in helping me create a new life in a new place because she adapted quickly—a dog is wherever the bowls of food and water are—and she was a magnet that drew people to us. I bought a new bike, a beach cruiser, and often rode around on it, which made me feel youthful. I took a lot of walks, opened up my mind and heart, and started meeting people. Soon I was loving my new life by the beach in La Jolla.

I've had so many starts that I'm like a faulty lighter, but if I can do it, you can do it, which brings us to the next section!

Healing Afterwards

Obviously, I'm all about moving on. That's why I titled this book *Next!* Don't get stuck! Always keep momentum going, especially after a divorce or breakup. It's going to take time to process your feelings. That could mean a lot of crying, talking to your friends, getting spiritual, going on long hikes—whatever it takes to draw strength into your character and open up your mind to a new relationship. But don't say, "I failed. I feel sorry for myself because he cheated on me." No matter what the cause for the sorrow is, don't wallow in it. Do not!

It's a natural tendency to dwell on the negatives and the pain, but it doesn't bring anything to the table. It's not good for you. Pretty soon you'll be running to the doctor for antidepressants. Tap into the love of your children, your family, your friends. Get out in nature. Do a lot of work on yourself. Take classes, exercise, try a new hobby, and change your hairstyle. Power yourself up. There are many chances to reinvent yourself. Take advantage of them!

Here are some post-divorce/breakup healing tips that will help you get over it so that you can get on with it:

Friends-and-Family Fix

Surrounding yourself with people who love you will help tremendously. When a serious relationship ends, people often want to withdraw from others because they feel dejected and lost. Though it's important to process what happened, I don't believe that crawling into a cave will help anyone. Humans are social creatures; we need companionship. Ask a friend to join you for dinner and a movie. Accept the social invitations extended to you. Meet your sister for coffee. Talk and bond whenever you can. Pretty soon you'll find that staying busy and social has helped you move forward to the next step.

Dog Therapy

I highly recommend getting a dog. You won't feel alone, and every day you'll be greeted with love. Dogs keep us happy, healthy, and active.

Bedding Down

I'd spend my last dollar on a bed as opposed to new clothes, because your bed is where the action is, as well as the recuperation. When I first moved to San Diego, I bought a big brass bed, just like the Bob Dylan song, that came from a movie set in Texas. I loved that bed! Likewise for you, I suggest purchasing an attractive frame, high-quality mattress, tons of pillows, soft sheets, and a down comforter. That way, when you shut your eyes you will feel as though you've found sanctuary. Then when you open those eyes one day to a new person between the sheets, you'll realize that there really are many "someones" out there for everyone and you just snagged one.

Walking Cure

Put on casual clothes and sunblock and grab a bottle of water. Walk and breathe. You'll feel as though you've gone to the end of the world and beyond as you see little movies playing in your mind. You'll revisit past experiences while imagining where life could take you. Walking is a good physical as well as mental exercise.

Relaxation Road

Baby yourself. Get massages and pedicures, for instance. If money is tight, look for deals on sites like Groupon. Take a bubble bath surrounded by scented candles and gossip magazines. Or share a lovely bottle of wine with a friend. Whatever your painless poison(s) may be, indulge yourself in ways that will relax and rejuvenate you.

Health Focus

Eat well. Exercise. Stay calm. Think upbeat thoughts. Meditate. None of this is groundbreaking new advice, but it's amazing to me how many people let their health fizzle out with their relationships. When you experience a lot of emotional turmoil, it is vital to stay in healthy balance (or at least try!) through nutrition, physical exertion, and an encouraging outlook.

New Delights

Find new places that invigorate you like cafes, restaurants, concert venues, and gyms and make them your own. Don't go to the places that were your couple spots; they will just remind you of your ex and get you pining for those days when the relationship was good. You've got to change the energy around you—to "break it up." Don't stay locked in your old patterns, because you need newness. You can't leave the past behind if you keep repeating it, so do things at least a little differently every day and venture into hobbies and activities that you've always found intriguing but never tried. For a bigger change, consider getting a new home in a different neighborhood. The idea is to create new pathways that give your life oomph and trajectory.

Open-Ended Plan

I know by now you probably think I'm little Miss Planny Planny, so this statement will surprise you: *sometimes the worst enemy you can have is a plan*. To clarify, you need to schedule girls' nights and weekend getaways and sign up for gym classes in order to stay busy and give yourself activities to look forward to. While I plan social events all the time, *I've never lived by a plan*.

People often think that they need to "stick to a plan" of where they're going to live and work and how they're going to raise their children, for instance. Plans give our lives structure, which is good, but too much planning can eliminate spontaneity and the ability to take in new variables and make decisions. For instance, maybe you think you love living in Southern California and would never want to leave. But then you take a vacation to Wyoming and are blown away by the craggy peaks of the Grand Tetons, the cheaper cost of living, and the down-to-earth lifestyle you experience. You return to densely populated, expensive, fake-blonde-with-hooters Southern California and you question what in the world you're doing there.

Listen to your gut! Why not move to Wyoming? I am not saying you should book a U-haul the next day and take off like a cowboy to the sunset, but why not explore the idea of getting a job and place to live there? After a major breakup or divorce, you can just wake up and a feeling hits you with certainty. Your gut is making a compelling case for change, so you go with it. That's the decision you make.

In my case, after my divorce from Rick I wanted a new start and didn't really know exactly what that was going to be. I just packed up and said

I've got to move forward in a fresh way. I decided on San Diego, but other than that, there wasn't a detailed plan in place. I'm not saying everyone can make decisions that way. There are also family and financial pressures that can curb spontaneity. But don't underestimate the power of your gut. Maybe after your divorce you get offered a new job within your company, but at the same time you find out about a lower-paying but exciting job elsewhere that sounds like it is tailor-made for you. Which will you choose? Your gut is telling you to pursue the invigorating option even though you might not land it. At times in order to feel like you are really living, you need to take risks. In a transitional period, follow your gut feelings and make decisions on a day-to-day basis. Don't try to rework your life too much from the sidelines. Immerse yourself in the action and see where it takes you day by day.

The Lingering *What Have I Done, Not Done?*

Even when you're one-hundred percent sure that the relationship needed to end, you'll still grapple with gnawing questions after you've split. Let's take a look at those questions and how you can process and address them.

Was this the right thing to do for my children?

I don't think children should be a captive audience to screaming and hollering and general bad behavior. Children want to be in a safe, nurturing environment, and if that means the parents have to be separate from each other for that to happen, then so be it. I've never been one to believe that parents should stay together for the children, because they're making the children miserable too. The children witness what's going on and then grow up thinking that's what a relationship looks like. People can't fake being loving. Their true colors are going to come out and pretty soon a child is going to say, "What are you doing with Dad?" or "Are you okay?" Children are very verbal, smart, and observant. If things aren't working, you have to make tough choices and shouldn't play pretend.

I recently met a woman who said that she and her now ex-husband slept in separate bedrooms for over a decade and hadn't been in love for an even longer time. They stayed married because of their children. They didn't want their kids to grow up with divorced parents and to have to go back and forth between homes. Would I say that's a commendable decision to make? It seems to me that existing that way is a big waste of an adult's life. Plus, the children will probably realize it's a sham marriage and they'll definitely feel the tension in the household. I don't believe in making children daily witnesses of bad marriages. Moving on is better for you, your husband, and your kids.

How could something so good go so wrong?

You wonder if you had blinders on. Well, when we're in love we see what we want to. You might have dismissed the red flags that were there in the beginning flapping in the wind because you figured they would go away or wouldn't affect your life moving forward. Then lo and behold, those problems pop up again like groundhogs. The things that drove you from the relationship most likely were there from the start.

For example, a woman named Jenny married Keith, who was always coming home late on the weekdays. After work he would go to the gym and then bars and return to the house around 9 p.m. Though his behavior made Jenny feel like she was a low priority, she didn't think it was a deal breaker or that it would continue. Well, it was both, and they ended up divorced. But sometimes you truly can get blindsided. People can develop in ways that you would never expect.

Ask yourself: Were the signs there all along? Did I ignore them because everything else seemed solid? Or did something really change? If so, when and why? After you've gathered that information, analyze it, learn from it, and move on. Don't beat yourself up over it or churn it around repeatedly. We forge relationships with people we love; we have great times; sometimes it continues well and sometimes it doesn't. There is no deeper meaning that you have to uncover. Try to accept what happened and let go.

Why do some relationships last while others do not?

It boils down to consideration. When people consider each other's feelings, communicate with respect, and address problems together, they can then handle the stresses that come. For example, after having her second child a woman might feel like the house is too small for their growing family. Her husband agrees but can't afford a bigger one. If they both understand the situation, have a plan to resolve it, and act lovingly toward each other, then it sounds to me like they have a good marriage. They can work things out immediately instead of building resentment. On the other hand, when people feel that they don't count, that they haven't been listened to, or their goodness has been used against them, they reach a breaking point. Take a look at the consideration levels in your past relationship. Were you considerate of your ex? Was he considerate of you? Why or why not? Again, learn from it and carry on. Don't beat a dead horse.

Did I waste years of my life?

A relationship represents a time when two people came together who loved each other. Is that a waste? What would you have been doing otherwise? I like to joke with clients that the relationship took them off the streets. It let them share time, experiences, and knowledge with another person. In any relationship we grow. It's very easy to be single: to live by yourself and come home when you want to come home, eat when you want to eat. It's a no-brainer to be single. It can be lonely, but it's not hard because you're calling all the shots. In a relationship, however, you learn to be more open, adaptable, committed, and communicative—traits and experiences that are highly valuable.

If you stayed in a relationship in which bad behavior went on and on, you might wonder: Why did I deal with that for as long as I did? Maybe it's because you thought your partner would get help. You figured the behavior could get corrected, so you held on to hope and the love you felt for him. There are worse impulses. Sure, maybe you held on too long, but that can just be the way it goes before the relationship crashes and burns. Cut yourself some slack. Taking a risk with love is better than playing it safe.

Lastly, it's not productive to ruminate over having "wasted time" in a previous relationship because then you really are wasting time.

Am I to blame, or is he? Or are we both to blame?

I think our natural instinct at first is to blame the other person. "He didn't do this; he said that. It's his fault." But as you step back from the relationship and gain perspective, you'll often see in retrospect that you vowed to accept the other person for who he was and then made him wrong for it over time. For example, you knew when the relationship started that he didn't have much money or many prospects for changing his financial situation going forward, so the fact that you resented him down the line for not making enough money isn't totally his fault, right? It's not completely your fault either, in the sense that you're allowed to have needs and priorities that change.

I think the bigger lesson here is that there's nothing to be gained from the finger-pointing game. We're talking about two people who grew apart—who could no longer get along. That happens for all kinds of reasons, and there are no winners or losers. It just is what it is. I think if you're looking for someone to blame, you're looking at it the wrong way. Repeatedly blaming the other person will lead to bitterness, which will hold you back from moving on. Repeatedly blaming yourself is also self-defeating. Again, take your lessons from it and let go. Replaying what went wrong is not productive. You've experienced it. You've learned from it. Now what's next?

Finding the Next Love

There is no set time to wait before dating again. Some people put arbitrary timeframes on their single search like, "I must wait until a year after my divorce before I date again." Why? A divorce can take a very long time to process and prior to that, your marital problems probably stretched on for years. You'd been feeling single for a long time, even though another body occupied a home with you. My advice is to date when you want to. The right person could come along the day you sign your divorce papers. Be open to what comes your way.

This story illustrates my point. I was looking for female matches for a client of mine, an architect named Daniel. At the gym I spotted this gorgeous woman with olive skin and an outgoing personality and thought she'd be perfect for him. It turned out in speaking with Elena that she was married, but unhappily. When I told her about my match-making business and client Daniel, Elena opened up to me about her marital troubles and how her husband had instilled a financial fear in her that made her too scared to leave him. I gave her my card and told her to call me if anything changed. I added that I felt strongly that she should meet Daniel; I just knew they could forge a great connection.

A few months later Elena called and said she'd gotten a lawyer and was in the process of divorcing her husband. She was hesitant to meet Daniel because her divorce wasn't final, but I convinced her that there was no harm in a shaking of hands and a conversation and that Daniel would be made aware of her situation. Well, they met and the rest is history. They hit it off, dated, and got married! He was a real love bug who gave her the confidence and reassurance that she needed to move on. While she was separated from her husband who was playing financial hardball, Daniel gave Elena a job as a receptionist in his office. Daniel is quiet and intel-lectual, so Elena lit up his life with her fun-loving, easygoing, family-oriented ways. They fulfilled each other in the ways each sorely needed. To this day, that is one of my favorite matchmaking stories.

But imagine if Elena had been resistant to meeting Daniel, and he ended up marrying someone else. Would she have found the resolve to finalize the divorce and find love again? Who knows? What I do know is the importance of seizing the opportunities in front of you. Starting over is hard, except when you're ready. When you're ready, something won-derful always shows up.

Remarriage

You have all of the dating chapters in this book to help you along as you go from your divorce or breakup back into the mixing-and-mingling singles scene. So for now, I want to move onto a different subject: remarriage.

Why marry after a first or second divorce? I get asked that all the time. As I've said before, getting married is the ultimate feeling of completion.

You went to the top of the cake, and now you get to eat it. Marriage opens up the door for you to have the freedom to be yourself. Instead of exerting energy chasing someone, you can focus on who you are because you have the loving, secure foundation of marriage underneath you.

You entered into your first marriage because you fell in love and enjoyed the person's company. During the marriage you shared amazing days together and learned from the struggles. You had children, opened up your heart and soul, and experienced many situations and emotions. You cannot put a value on that; it's priceless. Over the long term, how is it better to be single—hitting the bars and waltzing through your days with your self-absorbed habits? That's fun at times, but unfulfilling in the long run. Vacillating, running from one person to another, living in your one-bedroom apartment, and doing your own thing is safe. In my opinion, marriage gives you true opportunities to really live, stretch yourself, and explore. I am so rah-rah for marriage and serious relationships.

A few women have been clients of mine over and over again. I run into them periodically and they're still single. They'll date a man—even for multiple years—but they just can't get into the idea of getting married again. It's a trust issue for starters. It's easier to protect yourself by not taking a chance on marriage again. You can find the reasons you need to justify why not to move forward. This keeps you from getting hurt or cheated on or any other negative event that could happen.

For instance, I had a very wealthy female client named Sam whose husband had left her. I set her up with John, and they were together for three years. John, who had even more money than she did, wanted to marry her, but Sam wouldn't accept this. After that she dated one guy after another without allowing any of those relationships to get too serious. She never moved in with any of the men, they never moved in with her, and she always went for guys who had less money. That put her in a position of control and gave her an easy excuse to not marry them: they didn't have enough money. It was a bizarre, self-fulfilling prophecy.

You would think that money would give you security and options. In Sam's case, it has kept her stuck. She is the queen of the empty castle and keeps watch over her stuff. Why not move a king in or at least a prince? Live a little. Take chances. As I've already noted, women get fixated on their own personal things and habits: their homes, pets, and sleeping routines, for instance. They become rigid. The longer they stay single the harder it is to incorporate all of those high-maintenance habits and the other person into the mix and make it all work. It's important to keep an open mind and not get ensnared in the playing-it-safe trap.

People could say, "Well look at you, Barbara, you kept ending up divorced, so how great is it to take a chance and remarry?" It's true that I divorced multiple times, but I stayed in each of those marriages for many years because there was a lot of good in each one. I have no regrets and would do it all over again, because I can look back at all the experiences and life lessons and say without hesitation, "That was a damn good movie!" To me, that's what it's all about. No one is going to shake your hand for never taking chances. Would you want your tombstone to read: "She lived life with caution"? But I will throw you nervous Nellies a bone: If remarriage makes you too skittish, fine, but at least open up your mind to a long-term committed relationship. Don't try to keep things light for too long because you'll just end up feeling unfulfilled.

After a breakup or divorce, women can feel as though they've run out of starts. Your body and mind are like an engine waiting to be ignited. You just need the key, and what that exact key is depends on the situation and time in your life. But love—LOVE—that exalted, high-powered word—is often the spark and don't you forget it!

Some Parting Words

WELL, THERE YOU HAVE IT: the various stages, starts, and stops along the path of love. I hope this book has empowered you with the tools and mindset necessary to keep moving onward toward whatever the next step might be for you now and at future points in your romantic life.

Hold onto *Next!* as a handy-dandy, go-to resource for when you're looking for a relationship, in one, or exiting one. In six months if you find yourself newly divorced after being married for ten years, for instance, brush up on the dating tips in the beginning of the book. Or, if you're ready to start trying for children, reexamine chapter twelve. When your marriage starts to feel a little lackluster, reread chapter eleven on keeping a marriage exciting. I also recommend casually placing the book in front of your unsuspecting partner so that he knows he's going to have to shape up or ship out!

Use *Next!* to help other women, like daughters, friends, and colleagues, through the difficult times they face in dating and relationships. Too often women will judge and compete with each other instead of showing compassion. We can all use a friend, especially when relationship troubles bring us down. So be kind and considerate of your fellow woman. Likewise, treat the men in your life with respect! They are just as hungry for and deserving of love as we are. If I could state in a handful of words the main message of this book, it would be to love yourself and others. This sounds simple, but it carries profound potential for improving your life and the lives of others.

You have the strength within you to create a wonderful life for yourself and the people you care about. And now you have valuable knowledge about how to handle relationship choices and challenges. Put that strength and knowledge together to be unstoppable in your pursuit of love! Take care of your health, explore new hobbies, and make lifestyle adjustments that show you care about your future. Put the dating back into your marriage. Whirl yourself through the revolving door if it's time to move on to a better match. Don't settle. Live. Don't regret. Learn. Don't suffer—heal! Think positive thoughts. Create momentum. Embrace an outlook of *next* and you will be rewarded!

Good Match
Assessment Lists

The Dream Match List

(see Chapter 3: The List: Creating Your Dream Match)

Must-Have List

1.

2.

3.

4.

5.

Wish List

1.

2.

3.

4.

5.

Deal Breakers

1.

2.

3.

4.

5.

First-Phase Test
(Three- or Four-Month Relationship Marker)
(see Chapter 8: Forward or Not? You Can't Change That)

1. How do you feel?

2. Are your active/inactive levels balanced?

3. Does he handle money well and is he generous with it?

4. Are your diet and daily habits an easy match?

5. Do you complement/complete each other?

6. How is his temperament?

7. Is he a good sexual match?

8. Does he have the gift of gab?

9. What are his friends like?

10. For single parents, does he pass the kid test?

11. How is he while out of his element?

12. Are your future goals aligned?

The Marriage Practicality Checklist

(see chapter 10: Trust Your Heart: The Marriage Leap)

Here's a quick, ten-point list of questions to ask yourself before getting married.

Circle "Yes" or "No," and then jot down any concerns, questions, or other comments.

1. Do you love him?
   Yes   No

2. Do you think he'll continue to be a good fit for you in the future?
   Yes   No

3. Do you have similar goals (regarding children, education, career, buying a home, etc.)?
   Yes   No

4. Is he employed, financially stable, and responsible with money? Do you agree on who will pay for what, who will work, and how you will spend your money?
   Yes   No

5. Do you have compatible views on childrearing, religion, and politics?
   Yes   No

6. Do you communicate effectively with each other?
   Yes   No

7. Are you comfortable around his family?
   Yes   No

8. Do his everyday habits work for you?
   Yes   No

9. Do you enjoy many of the same activities? Do you have similar active/inactive levels?
   Yes   No

10. Does he have a life with friends, hobbies, and interests outside of yours?
    Yes   No

What's his score?
Anything than less than a 9 out of 10 should give you serious pause!

Leave or Stay?

Checking the Indicators for Moving On or Not

(see chapter 13: Leave or Stay?)

In the categories below, write down any applicable information. Once you're finished, weigh the good with the bad. What picture of your relationship has formed?

Reasons to Stay

Must-Have Requirements Met

1.

2.

3.

4.

5.

Wish List Fulfillments

1.

2.

3.

4.

5.

Reasons to Leave

Concerns (which you may or may not be able to correct)

1.

2.

3.

4.

5.

Deal Breakers

(One is too many!)

Are there any? If so, what are they? Don't be afraid to be honest with yourself!

About the Authors

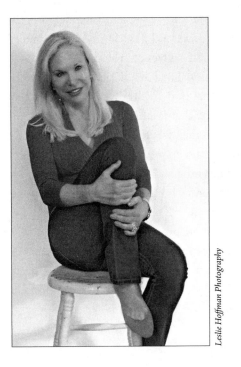

Leslie Hoffman Photography

Barbara Summers

Since launching her professional matchmaking business called Healthy Professional Singles in 1986, Barbara has matched over 300 couples who married.

Barbara also works as a relationship coach and leads seminars and workshops on topics such as how to keep a relationship hot, handling a divorce, and identifying what you're looking for in a partner. She hosts yearly retreats to Canyon Ranch.

Barbara is a proven media veteran, particularly as a relationship expert taking live call-ins. She has extensive experience as a live radio show host, including the *Bab Summers Show* on WJBK broadcasting out of Detroit and *Singles Talk* on San Diego's KCEO-AM (1000), which was a popular listener call-in program about relationships.

She recently appeared on *The Romance*, a reality TV series about dating that aired on San Diego Channel 4 and was nationally syndicated. Barbara has been a guest on other television programs such as *Good Morning San Diego*, *Fox 5 Morning News*, and Channels 7 (NBC) and 10 (ABC) San Diego evening news, and was featured in an Emmy Award–nominated documentary about the wives of professional athletes.

Prior to professional matchmaking, Barbara founded and ran companies called Love That Body (a fitness center), Love That Maid (a cleaning business), and Love That Job (a personnel agency). She has a passion for putting people together, whether it is for the purpose of employment or romance. Barbara studied psychology at Southern Illinois University and is passionate about fitness and health.

A relevant credential for the subject at hand is the fact that Barbara has been married four times. Yes, you read that right: four! (Note that the fourth is still in the picture, and his nickname is Lucky.) One of her husbands was a professional baseball player; another was a professional football player. She has a daughter, three stepsons, five grandchildren, and an Australian Labradoodle that is like an additional child in the family. Barbara lives in the San Diego area.

Carey Blakely

Carey is an author and freelance writer. In addition to various client work, she is currently writing a novel.

She is the co-author of *Crazy Like a Fox: One Principal's Triumph in the Inner City* by Dr. Ben Chavis with Carey Blakely, which was published by New American Library, a division of Penguin.

Carey has additional experience as a ghostwriter, freelance reporter, editor, and poet. She has also worked as a teacher and charter-school principal, among other jobs. She graduated early from UC Berkeley in 2001 with high academic distinction and a B.A. in English. Carey got engaged while writing *Next!* and now lives with her husband in the San Diego area.